Data-Driven Diagnostics

A Customer-Centric Approach to Healthcare Delivery

DR. SUMAN AGARWAL

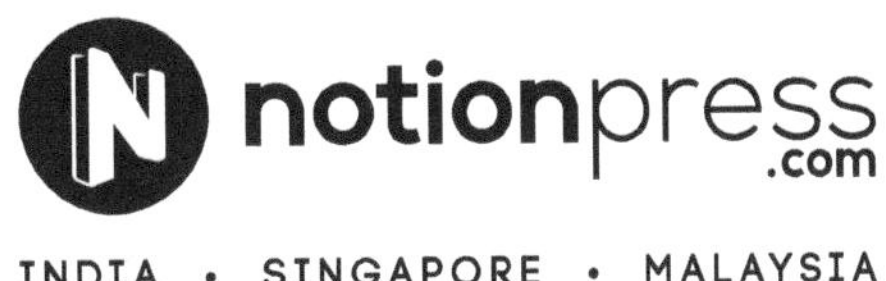
notionpress.com

INDIA • SINGAPORE • MALAYSIA

ISBN
Hardcase 979-8-89929-271-2
Paperback 979-8-89777-361-9

Table of Contents

List of Tables

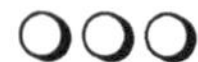

List of Figures

❍❍❍

List of Equations

❍❍❍

List of Abbreviations

CAGR	Compound Annual Growth Rate
ET	Economic Times
COVID	Coronavirus disease
CEM	Customer Experience Management
PAD	Pleasure, Arousal and Dominance
EXQ	Experience quality
CX	Customer Experience
SERVQUAL	Service Quality
RATER	Reliability, Assurance, Tangibles, Empathy, and Responsiveness
SERVPERF	Service Performance
GAP	Global Accountability Project
TCE	Total Customer Experience
TQS	Total Quality Service
TQM	Total Quality Management
NABL	National Accreditation Board for Testing and Calibration Laboratories
RQ	Research Question
ASEAN	Association of Southeast Asian Nations
SPSS	Statistical Package for the Social Sciences
KMO	Kaiser–Meyer–Olkin
SNA	Social Network Analysis

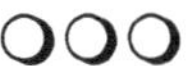

Preface

In the realm of healthcare, diagnostics stand as the cornerstone of effective disease management and treatment. The accuracy and timeliness of diagnostic services can significantly influence patient outcomes, making the quality of these services a critical concern for both patients and healthcare providers. This book delves into the intricate relationship between customer experience, service quality, and accountability within diagnostic centres, aiming to shed light on the multifaceted challenges and opportunities that exist in this vital sector.

The impetus for this book stems from the recognition that, despite the pivotal role diagnostic centres play in healthcare delivery, there remains a significant gap in our understanding of how these services are perceived by the very individuals they are meant to serve— the patients. The COVID-19 pandemic has further underscored the need for a more patient-centric approach in healthcare, prompting a re-evaluation of how diagnostic centres can better meet the evolving needs and expectations of their customers.

This book is the culmination of extensive research conducted in Guwahati, India, where we sought to uncover the lived experiences of diagnostic centre customers. Through a combination of data mining techniques and empirical surveys, we have endeavoured to provide a comprehensive overview of the factors that shape customer experience, service quality, and accountability in diagnostic centres. Our findings reveal both the strengths and weaknesses of the current diagnostic service landscape, offering actionable insights for healthcare providers, policymakers, and researchers alike.

The book is organized into five chapters, each building upon the previous one to present a holistic view of the subject matter. Chapter 1 introduces the reader to the importance of diagnostics in healthcare and outlines the objectives and significance of our study. Chapter 2 provides a thorough review of the existing literature, highlighting the gaps that our research aims to fill. Chapter 3 details the research design and methodology employed in our study, ensuring transparency and replicability. Chapter 4 presents the analysis and interpretation of our findings, offering a nuanced understanding of the complex interplay between customer experience, service quality, and accountability. Finally, Chapter 5 concludes the book by summarizing the key findings, discussing their implications, and suggesting avenues for future research.

We hope that this book will serve as a valuable resource for those interested in enhancing the quality of diagnostic services and improving patient satisfaction. By focusing on the customer's perspective, we aim to contribute to the broader discourse on healthcare quality and accountability, ultimately advocating for a more patient-centric approach in the diagnostic sector. It is our belief that by prioritizing the needs and experiences of patients, we can pave the way for a more accountable, efficient, and effective healthcare system.

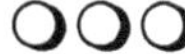

Acknowledgement

First and foremost, I am extremely grateful to my supervisor, Prof. Ranjit Singh, for his invaluable advice, continuous support, and unwavering patience throughout the writing of this book. His profound knowledge and extensive experience have been a constant source of inspiration and guidance during my academic research and in my daily life. His mentorship has been instrumental in shaping my understanding and approach to this complex and critical area of study.

I would also like to extend my heartfelt thanks to my friends and co-scholars—Dr. Banani Basistha, Dr. Bhartrihari Pandiya, Dr. Chandra Kant Upadhyay, Kajol, Lokendra Puri, and Lata Pandey. Their technical expertise and moral support have been invaluable, making my research and writing journey both enriching and enjoyable. Their contributions have significantly enhanced the quality and depth of this work.

Special thanks go to my interns and students—Aditya Raj, Nabarun, Prasurjya, and Ogchoy—for their dedication and hard work. Their contributions to my research have been essential, and their enthusiasm and commitment have been a constant source of motivation.

I am deeply grateful to my family—my parents, Mr. Mahabir Prasad Agarwal and Mrs. Shakuntala Agarwal, my husband, Mr. Ravi Agarwal, my brother, Mr. Saurabh Agarwal, and my children, Harshil Agarwal and Delisha Agarwal. Their unwavering support, understanding, and encouragement have been the bedrock of my strength. Their prayers and belief in me have sustained me through the challenges and triumphs of this journey.

Finally, I would like to express my deepest gratitude to God. Your guidance and strength have carried me through every step of this process. Your presence has been a constant reminder of the importance of perseverance and faith. I trust in Your continued guidance as I move forward, and I am eternally thankful for the opportunity to complete this work and contribute to the field of healthcare research.

– Dr. Suman Agarwal

❍❍❍

Chapter 1

Introduction

Diagnostics are a pivotal part of a patient's journey as 70% of medical decisions are based on laboratory results (Diagnostic-report-HLTH, 2022). Therefore, diagnosis is the first step to disease management, as without accurate identification, there is no possibility for accurate treatment. India's diagnostics market has experienced remarkable growth, valued at around $14 billion with an 11.5% CAGR (ET HealthWorld, Oct 28, 2023). This growth is likely to be driven by improving healthcare facilities, medical diagnostic and pathological laboratories, private-public projects, and the health insurance sector. The industry plays a significant role in the care continuum, be it for diagnosis, prevention, monitoring or treatment. The industry today is governed by forces of supply and demand, with service quality driving market success. Moreover, Covid-19 has accelerated the reliance on diagnostics and testing. The focus of the government since the start of the pandemic has been to scale and upgrade testing infrastructure and ensure the availability of testing kits.

Although some private providers in India maintain certain standards (particularly related to infrastructural aspects) in their facilities, the quality of care is not uniform; on the whole, it is often substandard (Phadke et al., 2013). Rashmi Mabiyan, (ET Healthworld, Oct 25, 2019) noted that the absence of regulation is putting pressure on prices, resulting in a lack of high-quality services and a proliferation of labs that do not adhere to conventional treatment standards, which compromises patient safety and raises questions about accountability in the healthcare system.

1.1 Modern Day Healthcare and Diagnostics

Healthcare systems are intricate, involving various treatment units, organizational functions, and departments that need to operate smoothly and consistently. At the same time, patients evaluate their experiences and feelings about the care they receive from these units. Therefore, building a strong partnership with patients is crucial for delivering outstanding care experiences, fostered by a culture that prioritizes service (Lee & Lee, 2022). Big data analytics and other advancements, particularly in the healthcare sector with digital health, have created new avenues for insight-gathering (Holmlund et al., 2020; Zainuddin et al., 2013; Skaria et al., 2020). Hoyer et al., (2020) has recommended that hospitals use cutting-edge artificial intelligence technologies to create experiential value. Clinical laboratories are essential to modern medicine in order to diagnose and treat patients (Hallworth, 2011). The daily dependence on diagnostics to make wise judgments is growing. Given the unusual COVID-19 scenario's high spread rate, it is clear that diagnosing and testing are necessary before making any recommendations that could save lives (Hosseinifard et al., 2021).

It is important to capitalize on the gradual transition in the healthcare sector from customer care to customer experience (Omachonu & Einspruch, 2010; Iyawa et al., 2016). Thus, one such less studied topic that needs to be investigated by the research community and institutions is the patient experience in health care services, particularly in diagnostics. This is demonstrated by the paucity of research on patient experience in healthcare and diagnostic centre quality (Swain & Kar, 2018), as the majority of studies overlook important aspects when examining and assessing patient experience.

1.2 Customer Experience

Customer experience is defined as the perception or acknowledgment that follows from the stimulated motivation of a consumer who observes or participates in an event which can enrich the value of services and products (Foroudi et al., 2018). Carbone and Haeckel (1994) described experience as the perception customers form while they learn about, use, maintain, and dispose of a product or service. They highlighted the cognitive aspect of experience. Shaw and Ivens (2002) saw customer experience as a combination of measured emotions and how well a company's performance matches customer expectations at every touchpoint. They stressed that customer experience involves both behavioural and emotional aspects. In a later study, Berry et al., (2006) focused on service clues in the customer experience. They argued that customers rely on many clues, whether they're aware of them or not, when choosing services or judging their experiences with services. The concept of experience is a multi-dimensional structure focusing on a customer's cognitive, emotional, behavioural, sensorial, and social responses to a firm's offerings during the customer's entire purchase journey (Gentile et al., 2007; Lemon and Verhoef, 2016).

There are certain researches which highlights the importance of functional capabilities such as behaviour of nurses, decoration, patient interaction, etc. in health care areas (Barnes & Mowatt, 1986; Crane & Lynch, 1988; Brown & Swartz, 1989). Worlu et al., (2016) presents three dimensions of Customer Experience Management (CEM) which are mechanic clues, humanic clues and functional clues. The significant relationship between customer experience and their satisfaction has been explored by Borishade et al., (2018) and found to be positively related. Santouridia and Trivellas (2010) confirmed this and found that these are very closely related. Adding to the research, Borishade (2017) added that buyers' psychological characteristics have a moderating effect on customer experience and their loyalty. In another research on hospital by Farhana et al., (2021), it was found that sensory experiences of the customer, their intellectual, affective and behavioural experiences have a positive impact on the equity dimensions of the customer like brand equity, value equity and relationship equity. To enhance this experience, employees have to cater to the unique needs of the patients and engage them (Reichheld, 2008). In a detailed study done by Ponsignon et al., (2015) categories and sub-categories of experience quality in healthcare were identified and suggesting a relationship between quality of experience and customers loyalty behaviour. For the healthcare service design, Lee (2019) proposed a model which can lead to excellent service quality by value creation. Kashif et al., (2016) revealed that two dimensions namely moments of truth and peace of mind and discussed how their customers highly value them as part of their experience.

1.2.1 Theories of Customer Experience

There are certain theories developed in the area of customer experience. These are given as follows:

- Mehrabian-Russell (PAD) Theory, 1974: It is based on the scale that integrates three independent emotions designed to capture information concerning the pleasure, arousal, and dominance dimensions.
- Chang and Hong (2010) have introduced quality experience model for service industries, which consist of five dimensions that are physical surroundings, customers themselves, service provider, other customer and customer companions.
- The four components of the customers' service experience (EXQ) scale—product experience, outcome focus, moments of truth, and peace of mind—were first presented by Klaus and Maklan (2012). Nevertheless, the entire quality of the customer experience is not measured by the EXQ scale.
- The definition of EXQ, or customer experience quality, was revised in 2013 and is now described as "the customer's cognitive and affective assessment of all direct and indirect encounters with the firm relating to their purchasing behavior." This idea is more pertinent to the caliber of services. According to Evardsson (2005), experience-related clues can be divided into two categories: clues pertaining to emotions and clues linked to functionality. There is a tendency toward functionality in the product experience and outcome focus. On the other hand, emotional experiences are more closely linked to the moment of truth and mental tranquility.
- Kim & So (2022) found that customer experience can be examined from three viewpoints: (1) the firm perspective, (2) the customer perspective (Chen and Chen, 2010; Pijls et al., 2017); and (3) the co-creation perspective
- The integrative understanding offered by Becker & Jaakkola (2020) is the needed step toward the development of a more unified customer experience theory (Figure 1.1)

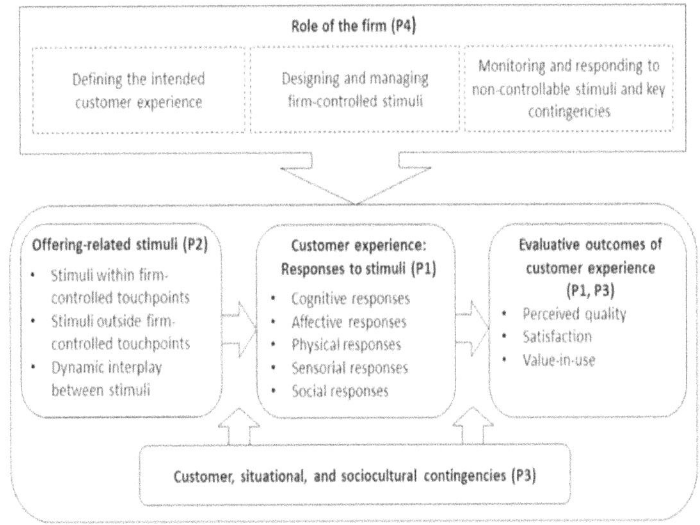

Source: Becker & Jaakkola, (2020)

Figure 1.1: **Conceptual framework for customer experience**

Based on the above argument, we believe that the customer experience in diagnostic centres should be measured at functionality/cognitive as well as emotional/affective perspective. Subsequently, the 28-item scale to measure customer experience in diagnostic centres is developed using findings from data mining study, literature review, expert opinions, and results of pilot study.

1.2.2 Customer Experience in Healthcare

The very difference of health services from other sectors is that the physical presence of the customer is a must as he or she is the consumer himself or herself. Therefore, the customer experience hugely depends on the service provider and customer interface (Garg et al., 2010). Health services fall in such category of services which are quite time taking and differ from one patient to other. But best health services should be provided to the patients and thus the customer experience is quite vital in this case (Farhana et al., 2021). In the healthcare sector of developing countries, the growing attention is on improving customer experience (Worlu et al., 2016).

The basic purpose of trying to understand the customer experience is to cater to the change evident from customer experience to experiential marketing which is a strategy for business growth and positioning (Garg et al., 2010). The ever-rising expectation of consumers in the health care sector should be met by the service providers. The quality needs to be improved because the patients have either kind of experience, positive or negative (Carbone & Haeckel, 1994). Baranova (2017) and Worlu et al., (2016) concluded that good and efficient delivery of customer experience acts as a benchmark and provides a competitive advantage leading to increased customer loyalty. Furthermore, understanding patient perceptions based on their experiences helps in improving the overall performance of the health care service providers and enhances the clinical outcome (Tajpour et al., 2020). The increasing rate of change in service delivery for consumers is forcing the organizations to think in this direction and implement by developing and strengthening their customer experience strategies. There can be mismatch between the expectations and judgment of the consumer with what is designed by the provider and so the seller's perspective shouldn't be considered as final and sufficient (Goldstein et al., 2002).

The literature in the area of customer experience showcases the 'customer journey' as the overall process the customer undergoes including the one-to-one encounter between the organization and the consumer (Voss et al., 2008). It is very evident that customer experience and interactions during the delivery of the service is very crucial while designing the service and delivering it after improvement (Baranova, 2017). Zolkiewski et al., (2017) proposed a consumer experience framework from a strategic point of view for healthcare organizations.

The customers in a diagnostic centre are the patients and ill people and they differ from the customers in any other organization. These customers come with a lot of anxiety, tension, stress, and negativity (Ulrey & Amason, 2001). Since customer experience is linked to cognitive and emotional functions (Kurtuluş & Cengiz, 2022; Jain et al., 2017), handling such types of customer needs special care and attention so that they can have a favourable customer experience which will lead to not only revisiting but also referring other customers to visit the diagnostic center (Ulrey & Amason, 2001). The customer visits any diagnostic centres and might have a positive or negative experience. If the experience is negative, it might lead to complaints against services. A thorough analysis of the complaints can provide significant insights into the customer experience in a diagnostic centre.

In the customer-centric era, customers represent a valuable source of ideas for improvements of care services based on their experiences, which may influence their decision to revisit or recommend healthcare providers through word-of-mouth (Lee, 2018). Healthcare organizations strive to provide excellent service experience to customers, as such experience is critical to the quality-of-care differentiation (Wolf, 2018). Thus, positive customer experience is an integral factor for customer satisfaction and organization performance (Lee, 2018; Wolf, 2018).

1.2.3 Customer Complaint, Data Mining and Customer Experience

Customer can register their experiences on various platforms available either in the form of reviews or complaints (Kawaf & Istanbulluoglu, 2019). Reviews can be positive or negative, however, complaint is essentially registering negative experiences. Customer complaints are one of the determining reflections of overall consumer experience especially unfavorable experiences (Vel′azquez et al., 2010). A close look at the quantum of complaints shows that the number is rising unabated and there is a need to establish a comprehensive and robust complaint system (Howarth et al., 2015). Websites and consumer forums have also made customers able to register their complaints against any company (Mei et al., 2019). As a result, thousands of complaints are registered daily on the consumer forums where the consumers expect that their problems will be resolved. Due to the huge number of complaints registered online on consumer forums, the companies are not able to address each complaint effectively. The digitalization of information has increased leading to better data collection but on the other hand, it is very tough and challenging to manage it. Given a database of complaints having complaint title and complaint text, data mining needs to be done so that the patterns of complaints can be recognized and solutions can be designed.

Regularly collecting and analyzing customer complaints is crucial for improving services (Yahui Hsieh, 2012; Chen et al., 2012). This data needs to be processed to make it useful, which involves cleaning, analyzing, and modeling it (Satish & Yusof, 2017).

Research has shown that using data mining techniques to study the link between system issues and customer complaints is effective (Xu et al., 2018; Yang et al., 2018; Ghazzawi & Alharbi, 2019). Some studies have used data mining in hospitals but focused on different areas, like the length of hospital stays (Khajehali & Alizadeh, 2017; Baek et al., 2018; Ayyoubzadeh et al., 2020) or predicting hospital admissions (Graham et al., 2018). Additionally, Vianna & Wazlawick (2020) used data mining to forecast morbidity rates in hospitals.

Data mining tools can be used to facilitate knowledge-driven decisions by analyzing data in an automated and supervised manner (Moreira et al., 2019). The Apriori algorithm has also been enhanced in the context of mining frequent datasets and related association rules (Wang and Jheng, 2020). Srikant & Agrawal

(1995) have provided the algorithm which is used to analyze the complaint texts and titles separately for identifying the major areas in which the complaints are lodged. The frequency of different terms used in the complaints has also been analyzed to create word clouds to visually represent the most frequent terms. Certain researchers have particularly used this algorithm for data mining aimed at discovering hidden information and patterns from databases that are huge in quantum (Kurnia et al., 2019; Sun, 2020; Ndruru & Hasugian, 2020). Another popular way of analyzing such types of reviews is to perform sentiment analysis. Sentiment analysis classifies the reviews into certain categories such as positive and negative sentiments; good or bad; greed and fear etc. (Lin et al., 2022) whereas aspect-based opinion mining classifies the data into a more precise classification based on the nature of reviews and the one performed by enhanced Apriori algorithm is better than sentiment analysis in terms of providing more accurate and precise classification (Ozyurt & Akcayol, 2021). Apriori algorithm proposed by Wang & Jheng (2019) is an enhanced and optimized algorithm based on the transaction address index table for reducing the transactions. This algorithm also reduces the number of candidate-sets and is more efficient. The previous version of the algorithm proposed by Agrawal & Srikant (1994) has to scan the database repeatedly to analyse patterns in the data.

1.3 Service Quality

Quality within service industries has been understood and defined in various ways. A significant contribution by Parasuraman, Zeithaml, and Berry (1988) was their concise definition of service quality. They described service quality as an overall judgment or attitude regarding the excellence of a service. They further explained that this judgment encompasses both the evaluation of the service outcome (what the customer actually receives) and the service delivery process (how the service is provided). Building on the ideas presented by Smith and Houston (1982) and Gronroos (1982), Parasuraman, Zeithaml, and Berry (1985, 1988) suggested that service quality is essentially the gap between consumers' expectations of 'what they want' and their perceptions of 'what they receive.' Based on this understanding, they introduced a measurement scale for service quality known as 'SERVQUAL.' This SERVQUAL scale has become a significant reference point in service quality research and has been widely used across various service industries.

1.3.1 SERVQUAL

The SERVQUAL scale is based on the *gap model* introduced by Parasuraman, Zeithaml, and Berry in the 1980s. This model suggests that satisfaction depends on the difference between what customers expect and what they actually experience. If the actual service is lower than expected, it is seen as poor quality. On the other hand, if the service exceeds expectations, it's considered good quality.

Gap Model

The expansion model of service quality was proposed by Parasuraman, Zeithaml, and Berry in 1988. They proposed five service quality gaps in this model. Service providers' inability to meet the needs and expectations of their consumers can be attributed to these five gaps. The explanation of this model's five gaps is as follows:

- First gap: misperception between management and customers. The management's ignorance of customer expectations is the root of this disparity.
- Gap2: The difference between the management's estimated and actual service gaps for customers. The unsteady market, carelessness, and lack of managerial resources are the root causes of this disparity.
- Gap 3: The actual service gap and service quality standards. When service providers fall short of management expectations, this gap arises.
- Gap 4: The lack of external communication and service delivery. When management conveys false promises to clients, a gap is created.
- The fifth gap is between the actual and expected services. When pre-service expectations of customers are not met by actual experiences, a gap occurs. Customers are satisfied if their actual experience exceeds their pre-service expectations. Customers are dissatisfied if their expectations are not met by the actual experience. Businesses must close the fifth gap in order to deliver satisfactory service because it has a favorable impact on customer satisfaction. (Bielawa et al., 2009; Almsalam, 2014).

The study looks at customer satisfaction with diagnostic services in the context of the fifth gap in the service quality model. Customer satisfaction in diagnostic services is achieved when the experience meets or beyond expectations. When an event falls short of expectations, dissatisfaction results (Magatef, 2015; Sadeghi & Bemani, 2011). Accordingly, satisfaction is indicated if there is no difference between expectations and experiences, or if it is negative. Additionally, if there is a positive difference—that is, if the customer is not satisfied—than expectations exceed experience (Figure 1.2).

According to the researchers (Parsuraman et al., 1985; Szymanski & Henard, 2001; Khiavi et al., 2018), when there's a negative gap (actual service is worse than expected), customers are dissatisfied. However, a positive gap (actual service is better than expected) can lead to customer delight. In simple terms, meeting or exceeding customer expectations can make them happy, while falling short can make them unhappy. The gap between perceived and expected quality can be well measured by SERVQUAL (Hamer, 2006). The SERVQUAL model, widely recognized and used, was developed by identifying and analyzing gaps in service quality (Figure 1). This model includes 22 statements grouped into five dimensions: reliability, assurance, tangibility, empathy, and responsiveness, (Parsuraman et al., 1985) forming the RATER acronym (Table 1.1).

Each item in the SERVQUAL model is evaluated twice: first, to measure expectations about certain services in general, and second, to assess perceptions regarding specific services and the service company (Christoglou et al., 2006). The quality gap (Q) is calculated by subtracting expectations (E) from perceptions (P), P-E=Q (Parasuraman et al., 1988). The non-weighted or weighted average sum of dimensions' evaluation serves as an indicator of perceived service quality.

The formula to express this approach to measuring service quality is given in equation 1.1:

SQ =Σ (Pij – Eij *Equation 1.1*

where

SQ = Service Quality

Pij = Performance perception of stimulus i with respect to attribute j

Eij = Service quality expectation for attribute j that is the relevant norm for stimulus i

In simpler terms, the difference between what a customer perceives (P) and what they expect (E) helps determine their perceived service quality. A higher (more positive) score suggests better perceived service quality.

Table 1.1: **Presentation and meaning of SERVQUAL dimensions**

RELIABILITY Delivering on promises	Your ability to perform the promised service dependably and accurately	• Timeliness • Consistency/Regularity • Accuracy
ASSURANCE Inspiring trust and confidence	The knowledge and courtesy of staff; their ability to inspire trust and confidence	• Staff competence • Respect for stakeholders • Credibility • Probity and confidentiality • Safety and security
TANGIBLES Representing the service physically	The physical representations or images of your service	• Physical facilities • Equipment • Technology • Employees • Communication materials
EMPATHY Treating customers as individuals	The caring individualized attention you provide your stakeholders	• Access (to staff, services, information) • Communication (clear, appropriate, timely) • Understanding the stakeholder • Services appropriate for stakeholders' needs • Individualized attention
RESPONSIVENESS Being willing to help	Your willingness to help customers and to provide prompt service	• Willingness to help • Prompt attention to requests, questions • Problem resolution • Complaint handling • Flexibility

Source: Zeithaml, A. V., Parasuraman, A. and Berry, L. L. (1990), Delivering Quality Service. The Free Press

The significance of the scale developed by Parasuraman, Zeithaml, and Berry in 1988 is clear from its use in many research studies across different service industries. This scale has been applied in various empirical studies in fields such as marketing, hospitality, and customer service by researchers like

Brown and Swartz (1989), Carman (1990), Kassim & Bojei (2002), Lewis (1987; 1991), Pitt et al., (1992), Witkowski & Wolfinbarger (2002), and Young et al., (1994).

As quality standards are more difficult to establish in service operations, measuring and improving service quality is crucial for a service company to reach its strategic, marketing, and financial goals (Lee & Lee, 2022). Ladhari (2009) agrees, stating that SERVQUAL is a reliable scale for measuring service quality across various industries. However, he emphasizes that the key dimensions of the SERVQUAL model should be tailored to fit the specific characteristics of each industry. Based on different understandings, several different scales have been suggested for measuring service quality. For example, studies by Brady, Cronin, and Brand (2002); Cronin and Taylor (1992, 1994); Dabholkar et al., (2000); as well as Parasuraman, Zeithaml, and Berry (1985, 1988) have proposed alternative measurement scales for assessing service quality.

1.3.3 Healthcare Service Quality

Apart from the favourable customer experience, another important factor for the success of the diagnostic centre is the perception of customers towards its service quality. Medical service quality can be assessed in two main areas: clinical quality and perceived quality. Clinical quality pertains to objective medical outcomes, while perceived quality relates to patients' subjective experiences, including how they were treated, cared for, and engaged with at a medical facility (Park et al., 2016). Positive perception towards various aspects of its service quality, such as reliability, tangibility, empathy, assurance, compliance, etc. (Parasuraman et al., 1988; Singh and Choudhury, 2017) restore the faith of customers in its services and results in satisfaction of customers and thereby bringing more customer (Bielawa et al., 2009). The role of service quality in the survival and success of diagnostic centres has failed to acknowledge its significant impact on the industry's competitiveness. In the health sector, enhancing service quality is now considered the most important step in gaining a competitive edge in the market. (Rula Al-Damen, 2017), patient satisfaction is an important measure of service quality in healthcare systems. Patients' feelings are crucial to improving services (Wysong & Driver, 2009). Patients' arguments are important, in line with the "marketing concept," which focuses on ensuring customer satisfaction and considering that patients are neither right nor wrong but satisfied.

Patients consume health services simultaneously as they are produced, making it challenging for them to assess service quality prior to receiving care (Babakus and Mangold, 1992). Healthcare service quality is influenced by the service process and interactions between customers and service providers. Certain attributes of healthcare quality, such as timeliness, consistency, and accuracy, pose challenges for measurement beyond subjective assessments by customers (Mosadeghrad, 2012). The unique characteristics of healthcare, including intangibility, heterogeneity, and simultaneity, pose challenges in defining and measuring quality (Mosadeghrad, 2014a; Naveh & Stern, 2005). Mosadeghrad (2014b) defined quality healthcare as consistently pleasing patients by delivering effective, efficient, and beneficial healthcare services that align with the latest clinical guidelines and standard s. These services should meet patients' needs while also satisfying healthcare providers. Healthcare's complex nature, along with the diverse interests of healthcare providers and ethical considerations, further complicate the matter (Eiriz & Figueiredo, 2005; Mosadeghrad, 2012). Additionally, variations in the background, experience, skills, and personal characteristics of healthcare professionals contribute to differences in service provision for patients (Joss & Kogan, 1995; McLaughlin & Kaluzny, 2006). These factors collectively make it challenging to establish consistent standards for healthcare quality assessment and improvement. Therefore, quality in healthcare should be measured from the perspectives of stakeholders like patients, providers, and managers, based on societal values (Padma et al., 2009; Donabedian, 1980).

1.3.4 Models for Measuring Healthcare Service Quality

Quality healthcare is a subjective, complex, and multi-dimensional concept (Lee & Lee, 2022). Different models and dimensions have been evolved and developed after SERVQUAL in healthcare service quality literature. There is still a need to develop new models, add new contextual dimensions and items in existing models on different aspects of healthcare services (Endeshaw, 2021; Ali et al., 2023), because generic models like SERVQUAL may not fully capture the complex nature of healthcare services. They often overlook technical aspects and cultural contexts (Alizadeh et al., 2016). Six main models are identified: Donabedian's, SERVQUAL, HEALTHQUAL, PubHosQual, HospitalQual, and Multi-level Healthcare Service Quality (HSQ) Model.

A. Donabedian's Model

Donabedian is known as the pioneer in studying healthcare quality. He believed that improving healthcare quality depends on both technical (medical treatment) and interpersonal (communication with patients) aspects (Donabedian, 1987). Donabedian (1987) suggested using three main items: structure (healthcare settings and qualifications), process (healthcare activities), and outcome (patient results). He identified seven dimensions to measure healthcare quality: efficacy, effectiveness, efficiency, optimality, acceptability, legitimacy, and equity (Donabedian, 2003).

B. SERVQUAL in Healthcare

The SERVQUAL method facilitates the provider to learn the patient's expectations and can identify irregularities to implement corrections (Jonkisz et al., 2021). This popular model has been used in healthcare despite some debates over its validity and reliability (Carman, 1990; Babakus & Boller, 1992; Sureshchandar et al., 2001). Various studies have adapted SERVQUAL to fit healthcare contexts (Al-Borie et al., 2013; Anderson, 1995; Kilbourne et al., 2004; Jonkisz et al., 2021; Purcărea et al., 2013; Chakraborty & Majumdar, 2011; AlOmari, 2021; Curry & Sinclair, 2002; Dean A, 1999; Al-Neyadi et al., 2018). Developed by Parasuraman, Zeithaml, and Berry in 1985 and 1988, SERVQUAL is widely used to measure service quality. It is based on the Disconfirmation Model, which proposes that satisfaction depends on the disconfirmation of perception from expectation (Figure 1.1). Ali et al., (2024) adds patient safety and medical professionalism to the traditional SERVQUAL dimensions. Herstein and Gamliel (2010) included an extra dimension related to private branding. Darzi et al.,

(2023) identified 41 different dimensions of healthcare service quality measurement. These dimensions were classified into four categories: servicescape, personnel, hospital administration, and patients.

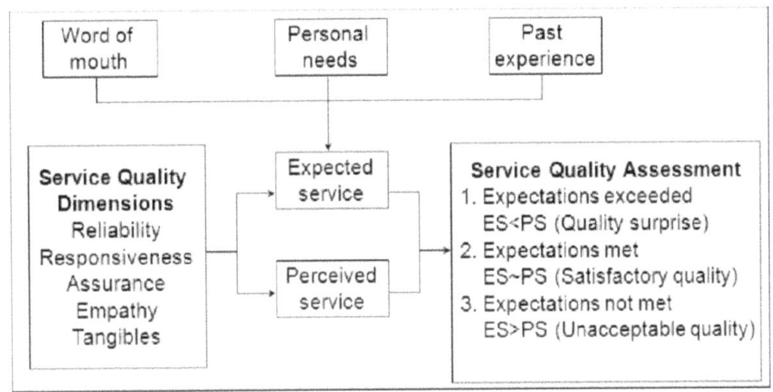

Source:: Zeithaml, V., Parasuraman, A. and Berry, L. L. (1990). Delivering service quality-balancing customer perceptions and expectations. New York: The Free Press.

Figure 1.2: **Expectation and perception in service quality assessment**

In summary, researchers continue to explore and adapt the SERVQUAL framework to better capture the nuances of healthcare service quality. Some studies modified SERVQUAL to better fit their contexts, while others argued for industry-specific dimensions.

C. HEALTHQUAL Model

While SERVQUAL is used in many service industries, many existing models are of Western origin and may not align with the cultural and economic contexts of developing countries. Endeshaw (2021) believed that healthcare needed its own model. Built on Donabedian's ideas (Donabedian, 1988), which focus on structure, process, and outcomes, Camilleri and O'Callaghan (1998) used this to create a model for hospitals in Malta. Their HEALTHQUAL model has six main parts: admission processes, doctor's attitudes, nursing staff's attitudes, hospital environment, patient facilities, and discharge planning.

D. PubHosQual Model

The PubHosQual model looks at public hospital quality from the patients' view (Aagja & Garg, 2010). It was made to assess public hospitals in India, using 24 questions grouped into five areas: admission, medical care, overall service, discharge, and social responsibility. This model helped identify areas needing improvement and was adapted as needed.

E. HospitalQual Model

Itumalla et al., (2014) made the HospitalQual model by tweaking the SERVQUAL model. This was specifically for monitoring and improving services for patients in a public hospital in Hyderabad, India. While it's good for hospital managers to improve services for in-patients, it does have its limits.

F. Multi-level Healthcare Service Quality (HSQ) Model

Sumaedi et al., (2016) have introduced a multi-tier Healthcare Service Quality (HSQ) model comprising three main dimensions:

Healthcare Service Outcome: Encompasses aspects such as waiting time, medication, and effectiveness.

Healthcare Service Interaction: Evaluates the quality of interactions between patients and healthcare providers.

Healthcare Service Environment: Focuses on the physical and organizational features of healthcare facilities.

Some researchers have only used general models like SERVQUAL and SERVPERF. However, there's evidence showing that many researchers have adjusted and customized these general service-quality models to fit the specific needs of healthcare services (Ali et al., 2023; Fatima et al., 2019; Lee et al., 2000). This research work has adopted SERVQUAL scale for measuring the perceived service quality of diagnostic centres because the study on diagnostic centre is first of its kind and therefore the usage of an established scale was found to be appropriate.

1.4 Accountability

Accountability and transparency enhance social relations. The typical view of accountability involves a governing entity (like government, regional health authority, or professional association) setting goals or objectives that providers or organizations must meet. Due to the authority of these governing bodies, providers or organizations feel obligated to report on their progress towards these goals (Denis, 2014). Regulatory bodies play a role in promoting accountability by maintaining professional registers, setting education standards, mandating continuous development, and offering ethical guidance (Mosadeghrad, 2014). Control systems are often designed primarily to hold individuals or groups accountable for their actions or the outcomes they produce (Mulgan, 2000). Accountability in this context means that individuals are rewarded for positive outcomes and face consequences for negative ones (Bovens, 2007; Priyadarshi & Kumar, 2020). These accountability-focused control systems are prevalent at managerial levels across most organizations. In some cases, they are also implemented at lower organizational levels (Merchant & Otley, 2006). Accountability in relationships means that an individual or organization is held responsible by another significant entity for meeting expected performance standards. Accountability can be seen as a series of challenges faced by leaders. These challenges encompass: assigning tasks and setting expectations; verifying task performance; ensuring responsiveness from those held accountable; assigning blame for actions; determining responsibility among various parties; identifying the ultimate authority; and navigating multiple accountability systems (Romzek & Dubnick, 2018). The three types of accountability are financial, performance, and political/democratic (Emanuel & Emanuel, 1996; Priyadarshi & Kumar, 2020). There are three strategies to enhance accountability: minimizing losses, ensuring compliance with procedures and standards, and learning from past experiences (Priyadarshi & Kumar, 2020).

1.4.1 Accountability Theories

There has been research work on accountability that led to the development of some theories and models in this area. These are given below:

a. The term "accountability" is used to describe a set of elements that affect conduct in social environments (Frink & Klimoski, 2004).
b. Accountability functions through formalizing expectations for behaviour or actions, establishing consequences for failure, fostering trust, and supplying the drive and incentives to use resources effectively (Cavill & Sohail, 2005).
c. Transparency, participation, evaluation, and complaint and response methods are the four elements that the GAP (Global Accountability Project) framework breaks down into when defining accountability. In order to be held accountable, a company must incorporate all of these factors into its policies, practices, and decision-making processes at all levels and stages of execution with respect to internal and external stakeholders. An organization's rules, processes, and procedures will be more accountable if they are of a better calibre and are more deeply ingrained (Blagescu, et al., 2005).
d. According to a Meso-level theory of accountability developed by Frink et al., (2008), which has been stated to have as its goal the prediction and control of behaviour, accountability is pervasive in social systems and is made more necessary in formal organizations. Deferring from others is a vital aspect of an organization, and this trait implies a blending of social and commercial activities, the people who make them up, and their various components, ranging from dyads to divisions.
e. According to Vance et al., (2013), distinguishing between accountability's two most common uses—as a virtue and a mechanism—will help you better comprehend it. Accountability is viewed as a virtue because it is a quality that people should exhibit when they are willing to accept responsibility. This quality is desirable in public figures, governmental organizations, or fictional characters. As a mechanism, accountability is understood as a procedure in which a person may be required to explain his or her activities to a third party who will have the authority to judge them and may also expose the person to potential repercussions.
f. According to a contingency theory of accountability, a variety of accountability mechanisms must be tailored to the needs and capabilities of the situation (Mansbridge, 2014).
g. The accountability hypothesis, developed by Vance et al., (2015) describes how the need to defend one's actions in front of a third-party drives people to think about and take responsibility for how decisions and judgements are made. As a result of this apparent need to take into account a decision-making process and outcome, there is a larger likelihood that someone will analyse their procedural actions thoroughly and methodically.

1.4.2 Accountability in Healthcare

With the increasing number and complexity of healthcare organizations, there's a growing need for accountable professional and governance to continually enhance clinical, operational, and financial performance (Glickman et al., 2007). Professionals must be accountable for the quality of care they provide (Mosadeghrad, 2014). No single model is appropriate to healthcare (Emanuel & Emanuel, 1996).

Health without accountability is a challenging task in hand, Accountability is the state or quality of being responsible, and it's a crucial aspect of healthcare reforms in India (Priyadarshi & Kumar, 2020). Accountability has emerged as a significant concern in healthcare, involving the justification and assumption of responsibility for actions. It encompasses three key elements:

i. Loci of Accountability: Healthcare involves multiple parties accountable for their actions or for holding others accountable;
ii. Domains of Accountability: Parties in healthcare can be held accountable for various activities, including professional competence, legal and ethical conduct, financial performance, access adequacy, public health promotion, and community benefit
iii. Procedures of Accountability: This includes formal and informal methods for assessing compliance with accountability domains and disseminating evaluations and responses (Emanuel & Emanuel, 1996).

Even though accountability is crucial for enhancing the administration and management of healthcare organizations and systems, it can also place an emphasis on learning and improvement rather than just control and sanctions (Denis, 2014).

1.5 Relationship among Customer Experience, Service Quality and Accountability

The success of diagnostic centres hinges on understanding and managing the intricate relationship between customer experience, service quality, and accountability.

a. Customer Experience Drives Service Quality and Accountability

- Positive customer experiences lead to higher expectations for service quality and accountability (Smith et al., 2017).
- Satisfied customers are more likely to perceive providers as accountable and deliver high-quality services consistently (Johnson & Clark, 2017).

b. Service Quality Enhances Customer Experience and Accountability

- High service quality contributes to positive customer experiences, increasing satisfaction and loyalty (Gong & Yi, 2018).
- Providers delivering high-quality services are perceived as more accountable for their actions and decisions (Leninkumar, 2017).

c. Accountability Reinforces Service Quality and Improves Customer Experience

- Accountability mechanisms drive providers to maintain high standards of service quality (Brown & Swartz, 1989).

- Transparent and accountable practices contribute to positive customer experiences, fostering trust and loyalty (Kushwaha et al., 2021).

1.6 Structure of the Thesis

There are five major chapters in the thesis. The details of the chapter is given herein under:

- **Chapter 1**: Chapter 1 is an introduction, and it presents a brief overview of the research topic, highlighting its concepts, theories, and major developments, key terms and concepts related to healthcare with special reference to diagnostic centres.
- **Chapter 2**: This chapter contains the literature review. A thorough literature review is conducted to analyse existing research in the area of customer experience, service quality and perception of accountability in the diagnostic centres. A thorough review of existing literature in the concerned field is done to identify gaps in the literature and highlight areas for further investigation.
- **Chapter 3**: Chapter 3 is research methodology section. The methodology section provides a comprehensive account of the research design, including the research approach and data collection methods. It describes in detail the sampling strategies and criteria for selecting the sample. This section is one of the most significant sections. Readers need to study thoroughly so that approaches can be understood. Ethical considerations and measures taken to ensure research rigour and validity have also been discussed.
- **Chapter 4**: The next chapter 4 is 'Analysis and Findings'. The analysis and findings of the study is presented under several subsection. Firstly, the findings of data mining done to extract the customer experiences on the basis of customer complaints is presented. Secondly, the analysis and findings of customer experience in diagnostic centres is given. Thirdly, service quality of the customers of diagnostic centre is given. The last sub-section, i.e., sub-section four contains the analysis and findings of customers perception of accountability.
- **Chapter 5**: Finally, chapter five presents the overall conclusion, implications, suggestions, and scope of future research.

1.7 Chapter Summary

Fundamentally, this chapter introduces the reader to the subject. It begins with a fundamental comprehension of the subject at hand. It discussed many aspects of the definition relevant to customer experience, service quality, and accountability in the context of diagnostic centres. It also discussed the various theories and models associated with the above concepts especially in the context of diagnostic centres. Following that, this chapter provides a summary of all the chapters, allowing the reader to grasp the entire study endeavour in one spot.

Chapter 2

Review of Literature

A literature review entails a meticulous and all-encompassing examination of established scholarly literature that pertains to a specific study topic or inquiry (Paul & Criado, 2020; Snyder, 2019). The literature review serves to establish the contextual framework and rationale for the research study. This allows researchers to structure their study in a manner that makes a significant contribution to the academic discipline. A comprehensive literature study serves to establish the researcher's credibility as a knowledgeable and informed scholar in the chosen topic by demonstrating their familiarity with the relevant literature. The literature review plays a crucial role in shaping the research design, methodology, and data collection methods (Kraus et al., 2020).

This chapter seeks to provide an in-depth understanding of the complexities surrounding the customer complaints, customer experience, service quality and customers perception of accountability through an in-depth review of the existing literature. This chapter provides an extensive review of the current state of scholarly literature. This chapter evaluates existing literature on customer complaints, customer experience, service quality and accountability in the context of healthcare in general and diagnostic services in particular. Finally, this chapter resulted in the identification of the research gap, which is discussed at the end of the chapter.

2.1 Customer Complaints

Customer complaints serve as a crucial reflection of overall consumer experiences, particularly unfavourable ones (Velázquez et al., 2010). By effectively utilizing customer feedback, organisations can enhance their overall performance and consequently improve customer experience (Singh et al., 2022; Satish & Yusof, 2017). Complaints can originate from former and current customers and should be taken seriously and addressed promptly (Cook, 2012). When analysed appropriately, customer complaints can be viewed as an opportunity to retain or attract new customers (Kiraz et al., 2020). Moreover, addressing customer concerns enhances customer satisfaction and upholds ethical standards in the marketplace (Campbell & Winterich, 2018).

Errors are inevitable in healthcare, and healthcare professionals should accept this reality. Acknowledging that mishaps may occur and patients may complain should prompt practitioners to develop a complaint management strategy (Howarth et al., 2015). Proactive mitigation is preferable to reactive complaint handling. Patient complaints should be viewed not just as post-consumption feedback but also as an opportunity to improve service delivery (Olsson, 2016). By collecting and aggregating patient descriptions of negative experiences online, patterns of poor clinical practice may be identified. Over time, this approach could help identify areas for improvement (Greaves et al., 2013). However, the internet is susceptible to false information, so separating reliable data from unreliable is crucial (Gandomi & Haider, 2015). Methods and analytics designed for managing and mining unreliable data must be employed to cope with erroneous and misleading information.

Complaint data should be comprehensively analysed to identify areas for improvement (Spiggle, 1994; Chen et al., 2012). Data mining techniques can be employed to investigate the relationship between system deficiencies and customer complaints (Chugani et al., 2018; Xu et al., 2018; Yang et al., 2018; Ghazzawi & Alharbi, 2019). While data mining has been applied in hospitals for various purposes (Khajehali & Alizadeh, 2017; Baek et al., 2018; Ayyoubzadeh et al., 2020; Graham et al., 2018; Vianna & Wazlawick, 2020), there is a lack of studies specifically focused on diagnostic clinics, which generate a substantial amount of customer service and complaint data. This research addresses this gap by analysing customer complaints from diagnostic centres.

2.2 Customer Experience

The customer experience is the result of a complex process involving company-customer interaction across various channels, influenced by both functional and emotional cues (Klaus & Maklan, 2013). Ferguson et al., (2010) also noted, the overall service experience before, during, and after the service encounter generates a value judgment. Moreover, sensory and social components of customer experience are included, making it more comprehensive. Value is jointly created when customers and businesses interact (Grönroos, 2012; Blasco-Arcas et al., 2014). Consequently, customer experience emerges from the customers' efforts to integrate and co-create value (Vargo & Lusch, 2008; Meyer & Schwager, 2007). Customer experience is defined by Johnston and Kong (2011) as the customer's perception of the service process and their contact and involvement with it during their journey or flow across multiple touchpoints. Johnson and Mathews (1997) found that customers who have had positive experiences with a service provider are more likely to have higher expectations for future encounters, while those with negative experiences have lower expectations. Carbone and Haeckel (1994) and Poulsson and Kale (2004) proposes that companies should focus on creating memorable and positive experiences for their customers in order to differentiate themselves from competitors and build customer loyalty. Haeckel et al., (2003) contend that companies must prioritize the customer experience to stay competitive in today's market. They propose a framework for managing the customer experience, consisting of four essential steps: (1) understanding the customer journey, (2) aligning the organization, (3) designing the customer experience, and (4) managing the customer experience. Mascarenhas et al., (2006) argue that achieving lasting customer loyalty requires a total customer experience (TCE) approach, which considers all touchpoints between the customer and the firm. According to Becker & Jaakkola (2020), firms should develop unique customer experience measures to capture different types of customer responses.

Gentile et al., (2007) provide an overview of the experience components that co-create value with the customer in order to sustain the customer experience. The authors argue that companies need to focus on all five stages of the customer journey: entering the experience, navigating/finding information, choosing, experiencing, and exiting. They also propose a model of the experience components that includes sense, feel, think, act, and relate, and explain how these components interact to create value for customers. The authors conclude that by focusing on these components and understanding how they co-create value with the customer, companies can develop strategies that sustain the customer experience over time. Ritchie and Hudson (2009) argue that consumer experience research should move beyond simply measuring satisfaction, towards exploring the broader range of affective, cognitive, and behavioural dimensions that make up these experiences. Verhoef et al., (2010) propose that companies can improve their business performance by focusing on creating positive customer experiences. The authors argue that customer experiences are influenced by various factors, including the customer's previous experiences, the company's internal processes, and the social and physical environment in which the experience occurs. Olsson et al., (2012) studied how customer experiences are shaped within the servicescape, the physical environment where services are delivered. The research found that these mechanisms are complex and influenced by cognitive, emotional, and social factors. By understanding these mechanisms, service providers can create more engaging servicescape, boosting customer satisfaction and loyalty.

In healthcare organisations, being customer-centric is the need of the hour to improve customer experiences, which helps in redesigning and expanding business processes (Schiavone et al., 2020; McColl-Kennedy et al., 2012). Customer experience is crucial as it serves as an organizational objective on its own. Additionally, insights from customers can be transformed into strategic solutions, facilitating the co-creation of customer value (Hudadoff, 2009). The customer's delight and loyalty are linked to a positive experience (Pine & Gilmore, 1999; Choudhury & Singh, 2021). It also highlights that a crucial factor determining the health care system quality is the patient's experience. Petersen (1988) opined that the experiences of the patient are more important even though the patient might be right or wrong.

Farhana et al., (2021) say that healthcare service providers can no longer ignore providing a better customer experience because of the severe competition and globalisation. These have provided various options to the customers and they are more aware of the issues relating to healthcare. This has created the demand for a better customer experience in this sector and thus, it has caught the attention of the service industry, particularly in developed countries (Worlu et al., 2016). Consequently, healthcare industry is focusing more towards automation of customer experience management (Safdar et al., 2019). Caru and Cova (2003) and Choudhury et al., (2016) explore customer experience from a marketing perspective, as the organisation aims to provide customers with memorable experiences. The customer experience is multidimensional because it includes many components like sensory, relational, cognitive, etc. (Gentile et al., 2007). User experience in the healthcare diagnosis journey, from parking to receiving diagnostic reports, involves a number of different interactions and experiences (Garg et al., 2010; Berry et al., 2002). Recent research emphasizes the importance of patient-centered care and customer experience in the healthcare industry (Fix et al., 2018; Coulter & Ligas, 2004; Nam & Lee, 2011; Weiss, 2023). Positive customer experiences lead to long-term relationships and improved customer satisfaction (McFadden et al. 2009; Payne & Frow, 2017; Greaves et al., 2013). Patients who are content with their healthcare experience are less inclined to seek medical services elsewhere and are more inclined to recommend the same hospital to others in need of care (Lupo, T. 2016). However, many healthcare systems priorities customer care over customer experience (Iyawa et al., 2016). Smart technologies can enhance customer experience (Weiss, 2023; Edvardsson, 2005), and there is a growing focus on improving customer experience in developing countries (Worlu et al., 2016; Klaus & Kuppelwieser, 2021). Prior research suggests organisations should utilise digitalisation to gather and analyse customer feedback for co-creation (Lenka et al., 2017). Alrubaiee & Alkaa'ida (2011) investigated the relationship between trust, satisfaction and perception of patients in healthcare service experience. They suggest that customer experience in the healthcare industry has a direct positive effect on customer trust and an indirect positive effect on trust mediated by customer satisfaction.

Given the connection between customer experience and cognitive and emotional functions (Jain et al., 2017), handling such clientele demands special care and attention to ensure a favourable customer experience. This, in turn, encourages repeat visits from existing customers as well as referrals to the diagnostic centre (Ulrey & Amason, 2001). An organization should establish the right culture, processes, and technical systems to ensure ongoing positive experiences for its customers (Smith et al., 2017).

Customer experience has garnered significant attention recently and is widely regarded as a crucial factor for improving favorable provider-user relationships (Yi and Gong, 2009), loyalty (Worlu et al., 2016; Klaus and Maklan, 2012; Smith and Wheeler, 2002), word-of-mouth (Klaus and Maklan, 2012; Weiss, 2023; Lee et al., 2012), and repurchase intentions (Verhoef et al., 2010; Lee, 2018). However, there is a lack of empirical studies examining customer experience from an integrated perspective in care processes (Zomerdijk and Voss, 2010; Lee, 2018).

2.3 Service Quality

The difficulty in accessing the utility of healthcare services places them in the category of credence goods. Therefore, even though the patient is the target when the services are being implemented (Georgiadou & Maditinos, 2017), the patient has a paradox when evaluating the quality of treatment obtained (Arrow, 1978). Service quality in healthcare diagnostic centres is essential for providing patient-centered treatment and achieving excellent health outcomes (Edgman-Levitan & Schoenbaum et al., 2021). Upadhyai et al., (2020) posited that in spite of health care being a professional service, the user defined service quality takes center stage. Agarwal et al., (2022), provided a research framework of service quality in healthcare citing several factors and dimensions contributing to healthcare service quality (Figure 2.1). Factors such as the physical environment, activities, and psychological experiences significantly influence customers' overall experiences and satisfaction levels (Xie et al., 2007). Donabedian (1987) advocated using a set of three interconnected elements, namely structure, process, and outcome, to assess the quality of healthcare services. Mosadeghrad (2012) elicited over 100 attributes of quality healthcare service and grouped them into five categories: efficacy, effectiveness, efficiency, empathy, and environment. Thompson (1983) considered seven dimensions for evaluating hospital service quality: “tangible”, “communications”, “relationships between staff and patients”, “waiting time”, “admission and discharge procedures”, “visiting procedures” and “religious needs”. Staff competency and training, effective communication, technological improvements, patient involvement, and process efficiency have all been recognized as variables influencing service quality in diagnostic centers (Zeithaml et al., 1988; Zineldin, 2006). Essential components of quality healthcare include appropriate technology, timely care, service alignment with demand, and maintaining medical practice standards (Handayani et al., 2015). Mulyana et al., (2017) found that the experience shaped by service quality dimensions—such as physical aspects, reliability, encounters, processes, and policies—significantly impacts customer trust. Johnson and Mathews (1997) highlights the importance of managing customer perceptions of service quality, and the role of communication and feedback in shaping those perceptions. Sureshchandar et al., (2002) suggested the soft aspects of Total Quality Service (TQS) – like managing human resources, focusing on customers, fostering a service culture, ensuring employee satisfaction, commitment and leadership from top management, and social responsibility. Seth et al., (2005) found that the outcomes and measurements of service quality are influenced by factors such as the type of service setting, the situation, time, and specific needs. Moreover, customer expectations for particular services also evolve due to factors like time, the frequency of encounters with a specific service, and the competitive environment.

Customers of diagnostic centres differ from those of other businesses in that they consist of patients as well as any family members or attendants who may be present. According to Ulrey and Amason (2001), these people frequently experience elevated levels of tension, anxiety, stress, and negativity. Within the constraints of the resources at their disposal, they must be pleased with the calibre of medical care received (Vogus & McClelland, 2016). Additionally, healthcare quality is crucial for business success, enabling customer base expansion, competitive advantage, and long-term profitability (Lee & Yoon, 2017; Handayani et al., 2015). According to Dagger and Sweeney (2007), service providers are placing a greater emphasis on service quality to gain market leadership as a result of the fierce rivalry in the services sector. Johnson and Mathews (1997) suggest that service providers should aim to consistently deliver high-quality service in order to meet or exceed customer expectations and build customer loyalty.

Service quality evolved from the Total Quality Management (TQM) movement of the 1980s but is hindered by its emphasis on the provider rather than the value received by customers (Klaus & Maklan, 2013). Leading experts who have researched quality for over 30 years include Crosby (1979), Deming (1986), and Juran and Godfrey (1988). Crosby (1979) defined quality as “conformance to requirements.” Deming (1986) did not provide a single definition of quality, but emphasized that quality is defined by the customer, stating that “the difficulty in defining quality is to translate future needs of the user into measurable characteristics, so that a product can be designed and turned out to give satisfaction at a price that the user will pay.” Juran (1988) described quality as “fitness for use.”

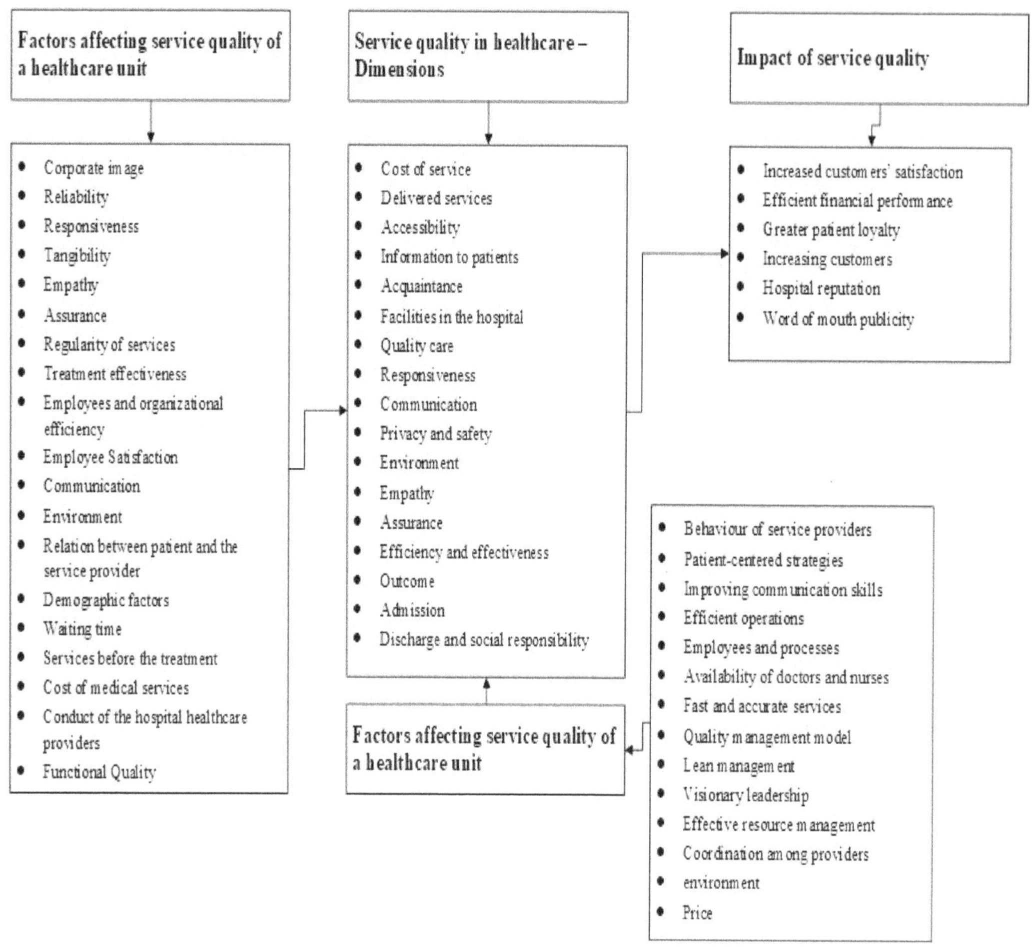

Source: Agarwal et al., 2022

***Figure 2.1:* Research Framework of Service Quality in the Area of Healthcare**

Additionally, Grönroos posits that both technical and functional quality are crucial for the success of service organizations. In healthcare, technical quality refers to the accuracy of diagnoses and procedures, while functional quality pertains to the delivery of healthcare services (Sohail, 2003). Measuring quality in healthcare is particularly challenging because it involves assessing the patient's health and quality of life (Pai & Chary, 2013). Johnston and Clark (2005) further argue that service quality is determined by the customer's experience and impression of the service experience.

Parasuraman, Zeithaml, and Berry (1985, 1988) introduced the concept of service quality, defining it as the variance between consumer expectations ('what they want') and their perceptions of the actual service received ('what they get'). Building on this idea, they developed a measurement scale for service quality known as 'SERVQUAL', often referred to as the "gaps model" or the SERVQUAL scale for measuring service quality (Parasuraman et al., 1988, 1991b). The model employs a 22-item scale to measure various service quality determinants. In this framework, customer satisfaction is characterized as the perceived service quality, representing the difference between the expected service and the perception of the service actually received (Parasuraman et al., 1985). Thus, the gap between perceived performance and expectations can be measured as a perceived service quality measure. As a result, if actual results exceed expectations, the consumer will be deemed satisfied;

however, if actual results fall short of expectations, the consumer will be deemed unsatisfied (Myers 2012, p.1; Szymanski & Henard, 2001). Another framework, SERVPERF, was developed by Cronin and Taylor (1994) using the same dimensions as SERVQUAL. SERVQUAL dimensions are used to measure the quality of healthcare services, besides additional sector-specific characteristics (Singh & Dixit, 2020).

Psomas and Jaca (2016) emphasized that organizations should prioritize a customer-focused culture to meet and exceed customer expectations, ensuring their satisfaction. Thus, for health service providers, measuring the critical factors contributing to customer satisfaction is a major concern. This assessment is essential for understanding and improving patient experiences and outcomes (Safdar et al., 2019; Psomas and Jaca 2016). This approach helps in understanding and fulfilling patient needs, leading to improved care quality and enhanced patient satisfaction. The equilibrium between customer expectations and actual experiences plays a pivotal role in determining customer satisfaction (Handayani et al., 2015). Measuring service quality and obtaining customer feedback on services enable the service providers to benchmark themselves with their competitors, adding value to their processes (Padma et al.; 2009). Perceived service quality is also likely to influence customer experience (Ismail et al., 2011), and as a result, it is probable that service quality will result in a positive customer experience. It is clear that service quality in healthcare diagnostic centres is critical to ensure patient happiness, trust, and positive health outcomes. Service quality dimensions, influencing factors, and the importance of service quality for patient outcomes should be essential concerns for diagnostic facilities and healthcare institutions (Ali et al., 2024).

2.3.1 SERVQUAL and its Dimensions

The gap model, first proposed by Parasuraman, Zeithaml, and Berry in 1985 and expanded upon in 1988, serves as the foundation for the SERVQUAL scale. This scale encompasses five dimensions: tangibility, reliability, responsiveness, assurance, and empathy. Widely adopted, the SERVQUAL instrument remains the primary method for evaluating customer perceptions of service quality (Lupo, T. 2016; Brandon-Jones & Silvestro, 2010; Wisniewski, 1996; Mohi, 2012; van Iwaarden et al., 2003).

a. **Reliability**: Reliability refers to a diagnostic center's ability to offer correct and fast results consistently. It includes protocol adherence, few errors, and quick turnaround times for test findings (Carpenter et al., 2020).
b. **Responsiveness**: Responsiveness refers to diagnostic centres' promptness and willingness to satisfy patient requirements and address issues. It takes into account things like appointment scheduling, wait times, and staff reaction to patient inquiries and demands (Ampofo, 2015; Hoe, 2007).
c. **Tangibles**: The physical components of the diagnostic centre, such as its facilities, equipment, cleanliness, and look, are referred to as tangibles. Positive patient impressions of service quality are influenced by aesthetically pleasant and well-maintained settings (Alolayyan & Alfaraj 2021).

d. **Assurance**: Assurance refers to the diagnostic centre's staff's competence, knowledge, and professionalism. It considers criteria such as healthcare professionals' qualifications, ability to communicate effectively, and capacity to provide patients with clear and correct information (Donabedian, 2002).

e. **Empathy**: Empathy refers to caring, personalised, compassionate interactions between staff and patients. It includes things like good communication, emotional support, and consideration for the patient's preferences and concerns (Duggirala, 2008).

2.4 Accountability

Accountability covers one party's guidelines and techniques to justify and take ownership of its behaviour (Emanuel & Emanuel, 1996). Accountability, also referred to as "answerability," is the duty to clarify and justify choices or actions made in public (Schedler, 1999). Three terms that are almost interchangeable and are substantially defined by each other are accountability, answerability, and responsibility (Elster, 1999; Schedler, 1999). Even if the idea of responsibility is becoming more and more popular both domestically and abroad, Schillemans (2013) and Bovens et al. (2015) asserted that it is still unclear and difficult to define. Instead of conceiving accountability as a problem to be resolved, it is to be seen as a process to be continuously refined (Thomas, 1998).

These days, healthcare quality, cost, and safety are all more crucial, with value (quality/cost) and safety serving as accountability catchphrases (Hendee, 2008). Any healthcare organization needs to have a suitable structure in place in order to promote accountability, foster openness, and support healthcare governance, all of which will enhance the quality of care. Responsibility is defined and practiced in patient safety cultures, and current research suggests that responsibility may have an impact on how effective healthcare organizations are (Bearman & Vokes, 2019). According to Priyadarshi and Kumar (2020), an accountable healthcare program and strategy will regularly review and restructure the processes to better meet the requirements of the patients and raise the bar for care. By avoiding professional complacency, moral responsibility upholds the patient's trust in the treating physician. Oftentimes, patients believe the therapist is working for them (Habli et al., 2020).

One of the reasons India's health services are not effective and efficient is the absence of accountability in the health sector (Das et al., 2016). Policymakers' professional accountability has been centred on raising the standard of care and making healthcare services more accessible in India. In addition, patient safety, transparency, professional responsibility, and organizational accountability must all be addressed in order to deliver the best possible healthcare outcomes (Kaini, 2013). The accountability mechanism has been impacted by the government's recent efforts to create an accountable healthcare system (Demirag et al., 2020).

Legal, political, and professional responsibility are only a few of the kinds of accountability that have developed over time and been proposed by different scholars (Romzek & Dubnick, 2018). According to Emanuel & Emanuel (1996), parties involved in the healthcare business may be held accountable for up to six different things at once: professional competency, ethical and legal behaviour, financial performance, access sufficiency, public health promotion, and community benefit.

In hierarchies within the health system, accountability linkages can be vertical, linking people who carry out tasks (actors, agents) to those who oversee them or are impacted by them (principals) (Cleary et al., 2013; Moncrieffe, 2011). There are several methods for obtaining accountability. While some focus on organizational behaviour and processes, others are more concerned with sanctions, results or outcomes, and reporting requirements (answerability) (Schillemans, 2013). Evaluating how actors, programs, or policies are doing in relation to pre-set goals or criteria is a common method of accountability (Brinkerhoff, 2003). An accountable business attends to the needs of its principal stakeholders in the course of achieving its goal (Blagescu et al., 2005). Employees need to practice more personal accountability and self-management skills because of changing trends and the makeup of the workforce (Dose & Klimoski, 1995). It is evident how crucial responsibility is when there is a lack of it, such as when promises are broken, criticism is rejected, or duties are neglected. Such accountability lapses have the potential to profoundly harm relationships (Witvliet et al., 2022).

Accountability benefits both the organization (by increasing credibility and legitimacy, strengthening governance structures, and encouraging learning and innovation) and its stakeholders (by ensuring that their demands are incorporated into organizational policies and practices) (Blagescu et al., 2005). The three primary factors that drive responsibility in the healthcare sector have been highlighted as being regulation, professionalism, and the market. Accountability may be demanded by patients, families, and other parties who are directly impacted by healthcare services (Pawlson et al., 2005).

Rabie et al. (2016) state that in the realm of service delivery, this implies that a service provider feels an obligation to provide good-quality services and, at a minimum, fulfils the terms of an explicit or implicit set of commitments to the patient or student. Furthermore, the provider is prepared to take responsibility for her/his actions. Accountable providers are more likely to exert the effort required to carry out their duties effectively, increasing service quality (Esther & Sara, 2015). The essence of accountability is answerability; being accountable means having the obligation to answer questions regarding decisions and actions (Brinkerhoff, 2003). Accountability, defined as the state or quality of being accountable, is a crucial element of India's healthcare reforms. Health without accountability is a challenging task at hand (Priyadarshi & Kumar, 2020). The ability of health clinic users to hold clinics accountable by exercising their exit option creates incentives for responsiveness and service quality improvement (Brinkerhoff, 2003). Ameera Shah (Managing Director of Metropolis) said, "The biggest challenge is the oversupply in the industry because anybody and everybody can start a pathology lab or an imaging centre without any consequences and this leads to a deficit of accountability towards the patients and the doctor." The competitive landscape for diagnostics service providers will persist, but service quality should not be compromised. Less than 1% of path labs are now accredited by NABL; under the Quality Council of India, certification needs to be more strictly enforced and the importance of high-quality services to the larger healthcare system needs to be acknowledged (Rashmi Mabiyan, ET Healthworld, Oct 25, 2019)). Brinkerhoff (2003) states that once the diagnostic centres and their employees are held accountable, they can learn from mistakes and continuously improve operations. A culture of accountability in healthcare improves service providers-patient trust, reduces the misuse of resources, and helps organisations provide better quality care. Measuring service quality is one technique to encourage accountability in the healthcare industry (Forster & Walraven, 2012). According to Conners et al., (2004), the foundation of any endeavour to enhance quality, form a cohesive team, and achieve outcomes is an attitude of accountability. A stakeholder who is held accountable recognizes the truth of a situation (perceives, sees, and relates to it), takes ownership of it, finds and applies original solutions to issues (solves it), and demonstrates the courage and commitment required to see it through to completion (does it) (Conners et al., 2004). All health systems contain accountability relationships of different types, which function with varying degrees of success. The perception of failed or insufficient accountability often furnishes the impetus for reform. (Esther & Sara, 2015).

It is the responsibility of a patient care system to compile valuable research data that can be analysed and applied to improve patient safety. To guarantee the process's success, organization members must be aware, attentive, and on the lookout (Boysen, 2013). Accountability rules and procedures uphold the unwavering idea that every employee in the healthcare industry does two jobs when they report for duty each day. If change-making is not made a daily, important part of everyone's job in every aspect of the healthcare system, it will not operate to its full potential (Batalden & Davidoff, 2007).

2.5 Research Gap

There exists a research gap in respect of the research in the areas mentioned above. The detailed research gap in the specified areas is indicated in the following paragraphs:

2.5.1 Research Gap in Studies Related to Customer Complaints

Customer complaints, data mining approaches for customer complaint analysis, and customer experience in the healthcare sector have all been extensively researched as stand-alone subjects, according to a thorough examination of the literature. Nonetheless, a large amount of the pertinent empirical research has been carried out in countries other than India. Although data mining technique has been used in many industries, there is still little of it used in diagnostic centers. In a similar vein, there is a dearth of study expressly devoted to analyzing consumer complaints to understand the experience that patients have in diagnostic centers. Despite the efforts of academics and commercial entities investigating customer experience, there is always room for additional scholarly research in this sector (Verhoef et al., 2015). The purpose of this study is to fill up these gaps by locating client experiences through data mining techniques. From the literature discussed in the previous chapter, we observe that researchers from outside India have conducted most of the topic-relevant empirical research works. Though many studies have used data mining in other sectors, limited studies have been conducted in diagnostic centres. Similarly, a limited number of studies have been conducted to analyse customers' complaints and find out customers' experience in diagnostic centres. Consequently, in order to fill in the aforementioned research gaps and obtain understanding of the negative experiences that customers have had in the diagnostic centres, it is imperative that customer complaint data be examined using data mining techniques.

2.5.2 Research Gap in Studies Related to Customer Experience

There are very limited studies on customer experience in healthcare. Also, a commonly accepted scale measuring the customer experience in healthcare has not been found in the literature (Kurtuluş & Cengiz, 2022). The literature research reveals that customers' experiences within the healthcare business have been thoroughly examined as independent fields of study. Nonetheless, there are two issues with the material that is currently available regarding the healthcare sector. One, the research is outdated, and the way customers interact with brands is always evolving. Secondly, research is undertaken in India in relatively small numbers. Thirdly, and perhaps most significantly, the research is carried out in hospitals rather than diagnostic centres. The diagnostic centre has not received much research in the healthcare industry. These holes should be filled by this study.

2.5.3 Research Gap in Studies Related to Service Quality

The analysis of the literature emphasizes the importance of healthcare professionals and administrators in diagnostic centers prioritizing service quality and implementing initiatives to improve it. While a great deal of empirical research has been carried out to define, measure and improve the quality of healthcare, especially in hospitals (Powell & Hannah, 2024), very limited research has been carried out in diagnostic centres. Not many studies focus on comparing the quality of these centres, so it is hard to figure out what works best. While we often check if patients are happy, we need more research on other things that matter to patients/customers who visit a diagnostic centre. Also, most studies are from Western countries, so we need research that fits different places and healthcare systems. There is no agreed way to measure how good these centres are, so we need better ways to do that. This study aims to fill these research gaps by empirically exploring the attributes of the quality of healthcare services from the perspective of diagnostic centres. Fixing these gaps can help improve how diagnostic centres work, make patients happier, and overall make healthcare better.

2.5.4 Research Gap in Studies Related to Accountability

In order to consistently enhance the delivery of health services, providers need to be aware of what their clients believe about their accountability. In order to pursue continuous professional development, which includes developing and retaining clinical expertise, analysing and improving care delivery systems, and taking part in quality planning, assessment of accountability is crucial (Witvliet et al., 2022). Customers' decision-making when selecting a diagnostic centre is heavily influenced by their perception of the centre's accountability. The subject of accountability has been the subject of extensive research. Nonetheless, research on consumers' perceptions of accountability in diagnostic services is still lacking. Additionally, there isn't a set scale in place at the moment to evaluate the level of accountability in diagnostic services. In order to close these research gaps, this study will empirically investigate the attributes of customers' view of diagnostic centers' accountability. Fixing these gaps can help improve how diagnostic centres work, make patients happier, and overall make healthcare better.

Therefore, any research effort undertaken to investigate the customers complaints, their experience in the diagnostic centre, their perception towards service quality, and accountability of the diagnostic centres would result in a significant contribution to the existing pool of knowledge and, therefore, should be considered as an important attempt to contribute and support the enhancement of healthcare sector significantly.

2.6 Chapter Summary

This chapter offered a comprehensive exploration of the intricate aspects related to customer complaints, customer experience, service quality, and customer perception of accountability by thoroughly reviewing existing literature. It delved into an extensive examination of scholarly works in this field, focusing on healthcare overall and diagnostic services specifically. Additionally, the chapter assessed the current scholarly landscape surrounding customer complaints, customer experience, service quality, and accountability within healthcare. Ultimately, the chapter identified a research gap, which was further discussed in the conclusion.

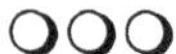

Chapter 3

Research Design

The importance of research methodology lies in its provision of a systematic framework for the structured gathering, analysis, and interpretation of data. Several factors underscore the significance of research methodology. A well-defined methodology ensures that the research process is meticulous, thereby preserving the credibility of the results. It outlines the steps taken to minimize biases, errors, and inaccuracies, thus enhancing the reliability of the findings. Methodology assists researchers in selecting appropriate data collection methods and techniques that align with the research objectives. Whether through surveys, interviews, experiments, or observations, the methodology offers a systematic approach to collecting relevant data. Reproduction is a crucial aspect of scientific research, playing a key role in validating and advancing our knowledge. A clear methodology allows other researchers to replicate the study, thereby confirming its results or extending the research in new directions. (Kothari, 2004; Saunders et al., 2009; Creswell & Creswell, 2017).

Research methodology ensures ethical conduct in research, with careful consideration for the rights and welfare of participants. Ethical behaviour in research methodology involves the proper treatment of participants, careful handling of data, and responsible dissemination of findings (Israel & Hay, 2006). Methodology provides guidance for data analysis and interpretation by defining appropriate statistical or qualitative methods. This ensures that findings are analysed in line with the research objectives and hypotheses. Additionally, methodology promotes objectivity by offering a structured framework for conducting research, helping researchers maintain a neutral and unbiased stance. It reduces the impact of personal biases, ensuring that conclusions are drawn from factual evidence rather than subjective opinions (Bryman, 2016).

A well-crafted research strategy optimizes the use of resources, such as time, funding, and personnel, by clearly defining research methodologies and objectives. Standard elements of research methodology include research design, data collection methods, data analysis procedures, and ethical considerations (Maxwell, 2012). Research design outlines the overall plan for the study, including the type of study, participant selection methods, and data collection techniques (Trochim, 2016). Data collection methods refer to specific techniques for gathering data, such as surveys or interviews. Data analysis procedures detail the steps for analysing collected data, including statistical methodologies or qualitative analysis approaches (Patton, 2014). Ethical considerations address issues like informed consent and participant confidentiality (Sieber, 1998). Overall, methodology provides an overview of essential components and ensures alignment with research objectives.

3.1 Statement of the Problem

The timely diagnosis of diseases helps in the prevention or the proper treatment of the illness. The patients or their caretakers, who are the buyers of health care services, screen the various available options to select the best possible diagnostic service (Wadhwa, 2002). The aim of the healthcare system is to provide services in a timely, safe, and efficient manner with equity so that it can be patient-centric and friendly (Worlu et al., 2016). From the survey of literature, it is revealed that health care providers are constantly striving to improve quality and efficiency by using performance management systems and quality improvement initiatives. Separate studies have been conducted to consider customers' experience, their perception of service quality, and healthcare service providers' accountability. However, a combined study considering all three aspects is yet to be conducted, and this study attempts to fill this gap. Moreover, the studies on the abovementioned areas were conducted on hospitals and other healthcare service providers but not exclusively on the diagnostic centre. This study also fills this gap. Therefore, considering this fact, it studies the different aspects of experience of customers and their perception towards service quality, and accountability of diagnostic centre and its consequent impacts on various aspects of working of diagnostic centre. This study is, therefore, customer-centred.

3.2 Overall Research Objectives, Questions, and Hypothesis

The study seeks to develop and design high-quality diagnostic service solutions, measures, accountability-strengthening strategies, etc., to improve the customer experience, service quality, and patient satisfaction with diagnostic centre services. The objectives of the study are summed up as follows:

1. To identify the items affecting customers' experience from their complaints using data mining technique;
2. To investigate the experience of the customers of the diagnostics centre concerning various dimensions of services;
3. To study the perception of customers with respect of various dimensions of service quality of diagnostics centre;
4. To study the customer's perception of accountability of the service providers.

In light of the above objectives, the following research questions are attempted to be answered in this study:

- RQ1: What are the negative customer experiences that lead to customer complaints?
- RQ2: What is the overall level of customer experience in diagnostic centres?
- RQ3: What are the factors influencing customer experience?
- RQ4: What is the overall level of customer expectation with respect to service quality of diagnostic centres?
- RQ5: What is the overall level of customer perception with respect to service quality of their diagnostic centres?

- RQ6: Is there any gap between expectation and perception of customers of diagnostic centres with respect to various dimensions of service quality?
- RQ7: What is the overall level of customer's perception of accountability of diagnostic centres?
- RQ8: What are the factors influencing the customer's perception of accountability of diagnostic centres?

The following hypothesis is tested in this study:

- $H0_1$: There is no significant difference between expectation and perception of customers of diagnostic centres with respect to various dimensions of service quality.

3.3 Overall Data and Methodology

Methodology is the detailed explanation of the essential procedures used to gather the required data for addressing the research problem. Research design is a systematic framework or blueprint that directs the execution of a research project (Creswell & Creswell, 2017). A research design encompasses the arrangement of conditions for collecting and analysing data in a manner that seeks to achieve a balance between the pertinence to the research objective and efficiency in the procedure (Leedy & Ormrod, 2023). The study is in two parts. First part of the study is based on secondary data extracted from the consumer complaints portals and the second part of the study is based on primary data collected from the customers of the diagnostic centres. The methodology adopted in this study is explained in detail in section 3.3.1 and 3.3.2.

3.3.1 Analysis of Customers Complaints to Extract Negative Customer Experiences

A close look at the quantum of complaints shows that the number is rising unabated and there is a need to establish a comprehensive and robust complaint system (Howarth et al., 2015). Websites and consumer forums have also made customers able to register their complaints against any company (Mei et al., 2019). As a result, thousands of complaints are registered daily on the consumer forums where the consumers expect that their problems will be resolved. Given a database of complaints having complaint title and complaint text, this study proposes to identify the major areas in which the complaints are being raised as a result of unfavourable customer experience. Thus, this research work is a novel endeavour that intends to identify the customers' experience in diagnostic centres from their complaints using data mining techniques. This research utilizes data from complaints filed against a prominent clinic on the consumer complaints website www.consumercomplaints.in. Analyzing complaints manually can be time-consuming and laborious. Data mining tools, on the other hand, can expedite knowledge-driven decision-making by automating and supervising data analysis (Agarwal et al., 2024). The Apriori algorithm is an effective tool for mining frequent datasets and associated association rules (Wang and Jheng, 2020). Researchers have employed this algorithm for data mining to uncover hidden patterns and insights from massive databases (Sun, 2020; Ndruru and Hasugian, 2020). Srikant and Agrawal (1995) developed the Apriori algorithm used to analyze complaint texts and titles separately to identify the primary complaint categories. The frequency of various terms used in complaints is also analyzed to create word clouds, visually representing the most prevalent terms. This study's primary objective is to employ data mining techniques to evaluate customer experiences at diagnostic centres. The customer experience database is derived from online complaints registered on the clinic's portal. Complaints were collected using web scraping with Selenium, BeautifulSoup, and Pandas in Python on an Ubuntu 20.04 machine. The dataset consists of 2096 complaints from various diagnostic centers across India. The complaints were collected and stored in spreadsheets having two columns namely "Title" and "Complaint Text".

A. Pre-processing of Complaints

The complaint data undergoes several pre-processing steps to clean and prepare it for analysis (Kanis & Müller, 2005; Wilbur & Sirotkin, 1992):

a. Character Removal: Unwanted characters are removed (Grefenstette, 1999).
b. Tokenization: Complaints are split into individual words or phrases.
c. Stop Word Removal: Common words with little meaning are removed (Wilbur & Sirotkin, 1992).
d. Lemmatization: Words are reduced to their root form (Liu et al., 2012; Plisson et al., 2004).

These steps ensure meaningful data for further analysis and modelling.

B. Data Analysis

The data analysis is explained in the following paragraphs:

I. The Apriori algorithm

The Apriori algorithm, developed by Agarwal and Srikant (1994), is a widely used method for frequent pattern mining, particularly in transaction databases (Grefenstette, 1999). Its key concepts and term definitions are as follows:

- Item: A unique object in the transactions database. In this context, each unique word in the list of complaints is considered an item.
- Transaction: A set of distinct items. In this context, the list of words from each complaint after pre-processing constitutes one transaction.
- Support: The total number of times an item appears in the transactions. It is often expressed as the ratio of the total number of occurrences of an item to the total number of transactions.
- Minimum Support: The minimum supports an item must have to be considered frequent. In this context, the minimum support of a word is the total number of complaints it appears in, divided by the total number of complaints.
- Candidate Item Sets: Item sets with a fixed number of items, often denoted by Ci, where 'i' represents the number of items in the item set.
- Frequent Itemsets: Item sets with support greater than the minimum support, often denoted by Li, where 'i' represents the number of items in the item set.
- Apriori Property: Any subset of a frequent itemset must also be a frequent itemset.

The Apriori algorithm employs a level-wise search to generate item sets. It starts with item sets containing one element and progressively generates item sets from lower levels to higher levels. The algorithm for generating C_1 is presented in Algorithm 1 given in table 3.1:

Table 3.1: **Algorithm 1-C_1 Generation**

Input: Data set with complaints as rows
Output: Candidate set C_1

```
Take an empty list C;
For every complaint in data set do:
        For every word in complaint do:
                if word not in C then:
                        add the word to C;
                end if;
        end for;
end for;
Sort C in alphabetical order;
Take an empty list C1;
for each item in C do:
        create a singleton set S using the item;
        add S to C1;
end for;
```

Source: Author's compilation

To generate candidates for the L_k item set, the L_k−1 item set is used. C_k, a superset of L_k, is generated by performing a set join operation on L_k−1 with itself. Algorithm 2 given in table 3.2 describes the procedure for generating C_k.

Table 3.2: **Algorithm 2-C_k Generation**

Input: L_{k-1}, k
Output: Candidate set C_1

```
Take an empty list Ck;
len ← length of Lk-1;
for i← 0 to len-1:
        for j← i+1 to len-1:
                L1← first k-2 items of Lk-1[i];
```

```
        L2← first k-2 items of L_{k-1}[j];
        sort L1;
        sort L2;
        if L1==L2:
            L= L1 ∪ L2;
            add L to C_k;
        end if;
    end for;
end for;
```

Source: Author's compilation

C_k is pruned using the Apriori property to eliminate candidate itemsets whose subsets are not frequent itemsets. Subsequently, the entire transaction data is scanned to identify item sets in C_k with a frequency exceeding the minimum support. Itemsets with support less than the minimum support are removed from C_k, resulting in the formation of L_k. Algorithm 3, given in table 3.3 details the process of scanning the data and generating L_k. This process iterates until no further item set with support greater than the minimum support can be generated.

***Table 3.3:* Algorithm 3-L_k Generation**

Input: Dataset, C_k, minimum support
Output: L_k with support count

```
Count← empty dictionary;
for complaint in dataset:
    Complaint_s ← Set(complaint);
    for candidate in C_k:
        if candidate is subset of Complaint_s:
            itemset← FrozenSet(candidate);
            if itemset not in Count:
                Count[itemset]←1;
            else:
                Count[itemset]← Count[itemset]+1;
            end if;
        end if;
    end for;
end for;
N← total number of complaints;
Support← empty dictionary;
L_k ← empty list;
```

```
for itemset in Count:
        support← Count[itemset]/N;
        if support > minimum support:
                add itemset to L_k;
                Support[itemset]← support;
        end if;
end for;
```

Source: Author's compilation

In this study, the Apriori algorithm is utilized to identify frequently co-occurring words in the complaint data. These frequent itemsets are then analysed for association rule mining to uncover closely related words in the complaints.

II. Association Rule Mining

Association rules capture the dependency of one data item on another within a dataset.[58] An association rule comprises an antecedent and a consequent. The antecedent represents a data item present in the data, while the consequent represents a data item that frequently co-occurs with the antecedent. The strength of this association is measured by confidence, which is the ratio of occurrences of the antecedent and consequent together to the occurrences of the antecedent alone (Zhang & He, 2010; Liu et al., 1999). Confidence values range from 0 to 1, with 1 indicating a strong association and 0 indicating no association. For this analysis, only rules with confidence greater than or equal to 0.7 were considered significant (Liu et al., 1999). Algorithm 4, presented in table 3.4 describes the procedure for mining association rules from frequent itemsets.

III. Word Cloud Generation

Frequent words were visualized using word clouds to represent their frequency in the data. Word sizes correspond to term frequencies, with larger words indicating higher frequencies (Heimerl et al., 2014). In this study, word clouds were generated from complaint data using the 'wordcloud' and 'matplotlib' modules in Python.

Table 3.4: **Association Rule Mining**

Input: Frequent itemsets
Output: Association rules with the antecedent, consequent, and confidence.

```
Create an empty set named rules;
for subset1 in itemset:
        for subset2 in itemset: #here subset1 and subset2 are mutually exclusive.
                support1 ← support of subset1;
                support2 ← support of subset2;
```

```
        support3 ← support of subset1∪ subset2;
        ratio1=support3/support1;
        ratio2=support3/support2;
        if ratio1 >=0.7:
            rule=(antecedent=subset1, consequent=subset2, confidence=ratio1);
            add rule to rules;
        end if;
        if ratio2 >=0.7:
            rule=(antecedent=subset2, consequent=subset1, confidence=ratio2);
            add rule to rules;
        end if;
    end for;
end for;
```

Source: Author's compilation

3.3.2 Methodology for Customer Experience, Perception of Service Quality and Accountability of Customers of Diagnostic Centres

- **Type of Study:** The study is descriptive in nature.
- **Place of Study:** The research is conducted in Assam, with Guwahati being selected as the primary data collection centre due to its status as the largest city and commercial hub of the North-Eastern States. Guwahati's extensive network of hospitals and diagnostic centres, along with its connectivity and strategic importance, make it an ideal choice for data collection (Deka and Devi, 2017; Haokip, 2015; Nambiar, 2018). Geographically situated in the heart of Northeast India, Assam serves as the gateway to the region's other six states and is known for its diverse ethnic and linguistic makeup, earning it the nickname "India in miniature" (Taher, 1994). Assam and its neighbouring Northeastern states share borders with ASEAN countries, and the shift from the Look East policy to the Act East policy has led to increased exports and economic opportunities (Sentinel Report, 2022). Assam's geostrategic location presents chances to expand trade both within and beyond borders, as well as to establish economic corridors between India and its neighbours in Southeast Asia (Asian Development Bank, 2021). According to Chandra et al. (2012), rising income levels also impact health-related decision-making, as individuals have more resources to allocate towards their well-being.
- **Data Collection:** The study is mainly based on primary data. The tool "interview schedule" was used to collect the necessary information. We have conducted a study to identify the customers' negative experiences extracted from the customers' complaints of the diagnostic centre using data mining tools. The data collection was conducted from February 2022 to June 2022. Customers were informed about the aim and purpose of the study, as well as the guarantee of confidentiality of answers.

Based on the findings of the first objective, the interview schedule was prepared to study the customer's experience in diagnostic centres empirically. Besides, the few items were adopted from the work of Choudhury & Singh (2015) and Choudhury et al., (2016). The result of the pilot study was also considered. In addition to these, researcher's own observation and experts' opinion was also obtained. Total 28 items were identified for scale construction for measuring customer experience level in diagnostic centres. A copy of the interview schedule is given in appendix. The responses were taken on Likert scale where the responses had the range from 'very favourable experience' to 'very unfavourable experience'. A score of 5 was designated for the response of 'very favourable experience'. Likewise, for the responses of 'favourable', 'moderate', 'unfavourable', and 'very unfavourable experience', the scores of 4, 3, 2, and 1 were assigned respectively.

2nd part of the interview schedule was prepared to measure customers' perception of the service quality of the services provided by the diagnostic centre. It is adapted from the study of Parsuraman et al., (1988). Utilizing service quality surveys to obtain client input is among the greatest methods (Zhang et al., 2023; Berry & Parasuraman, 1997). Service quality surveys provide several benefits. As they are provided right away following an engagement, the information is more accurate because it is still very recent in the customer's memory. They also provide information rapidly, enabling businesses to respond promptly to the most urgent problems (Engelhardt et al., 2020). The five dimensions-SERVQUAL model (tangibility, empathy, assurance, reliability and responsiveness) was implemented to measure the gap between patient's perception and expectation in health-care diagnostic service quality. Data was collected using a standardized interview schedule adopted from the work of Parsuraman et al., (1988) that includes 22 items of expectation and 22 items of perceived service quality aspects. The respondents were asked to complete the interview schedules on a five-point scale indicating their levels of expectations and perceptions in respect of various dimensions of the services of diagnostic centre. This systematic method permitted the collection of participants' impressions and opinions on several elements of service quality.

3rd part of the interview schedule was about the perception of the customers towards the accountability of the diagnostic centre. It was prepared on the basis of a literature review, observation, discussion with the experts, and a pilot study. To measure the perception of accountability, a scale was framed by considering 14 items. The language in the interview schedule was kept easy and simple so that the respondents could read it easily, understand it quickly and fill the answers. Copy of the interview schedule is given in appendix. For secondary data, official reports, records, Journals, etc., are consulted.

500 interview schedules were distributed, and 421 were returned, out of which 28 were found to be incomplete. So finally, 393 responses were used for analysis. The initial section of the interview schedule asks for demographic information from the respondents while the latter part targets to capture and measure their experience and perceptions.

- **Identification of Research Population:** For the proposed study, the universe consists of all those customers of different diagnostic centres in Guwahati city of Assam who have received any diagnostic services from the centres during a particular period.

- **Sampling design:** Sampling design refers to the process of selecting a subset of individuals or units from a broader population for inclusion in a study (Lohr, 2021). There are several types of sampling designs that researchers can choose from, depending on the nature of the study and the research questions being investigated. Some commonly used sample designs are simple random sampling, stratified sampling, cluster sampling, multistage sampling, and systematic sampling. Every sampling strategy has unique advantages and disadvantages, and researchers must carefully assess which design is most appropriate for the particular study. The objective of sampling design is to ensure that the selected subset is a true reflection of the greater population, enabling researchers to draw accurate inferences. Researchers carefully select the sample, a subset of the population, to precisely reflect the characteristics of the population. This allows researchers to draw reliable conclusions about the population using the data from the sample (Kothari, 2004). While formulating a sample design, it is essential for researchers to take into account various factors such as sample size, sampling frame, sampling method, and potential sources of bias. Researchers can improve the reliability and validity of study results by carefully planning and executing the sampling strategy (Hair et al., 2006; Cochran, 1977). The generalizability of study results to a larger population is affected by the sampling technique. Random sampling methods, such as simple random sampling, cluster sampling, or stratified random sampling, are frequently used due to their ability to minimize bias and increase the likelihood of receiving a sample that accurately reflects the total population (Levy & Lemeshow, 2013). Non-random sample approaches, such as convenience sampling or quota sampling, can introduce bias and limit the generalizability of study findings to a larger population (Babbie, 2020).
- **Sample size:** A sample of an acceptable size facilitates the conduction of statistically significant studies and the drawing of valid inferences (Saunders et al., 2009). Researchers can achieve a harmonious compromise between precision and practicality by meticulously calculating the sample size, considering statistical concerns. This approach guarantees that the study remains possible within the confines of the available resources (Krejcie & Morgan, 1970). For the calculation of an appropriate sample size several factors are considered such as confidence level, margin of error, and estimated population proportion (Cochran, 1977). In this study, confidence level is 95% and a margin of error is 5%. To calculate sample size, we have used following formula:

$$n = \frac{Z^2 \times p(1-p)}{e^2} \quad \text{...} \quad \textit{Equation 3.1}$$

Where:

n= sample size

Z= Z-score corresponding to the 95% level of confidence

p= estimated population proportion

e= margin of error

Given that the study is quantitative in nature, it is possible that we may not possess an estimated population proportion (p). Nevertheless, when calculating a mean or average value, it is possible to make an assumption based on prior research or pilot tests. Assuming a confidence level of 95% (with a corresponding Z-value of 1.96) and a margin of error of 5% (or $e = 0.05$). To estimate the population proportion, we will use a conservative value of 0.5, which will allow us to obtain the largest possible sample size.

Substituting the given values:

$$n = \frac{(1.96)^2 \text{ x } 0.5(1-0.5)}{(0.05)^2}$$

$$n = \frac{3.8416 \text{ x } 0.25}{0.0025}$$

$$n = \frac{0.9604}{0.0025}$$

$$n \approx 384.16$$

$$= 384.16 \rightarrow 385$$

Therefore, a sample size of 385 would be required with an expected sample proportion of 0.5 and a margin of error of ±0.05%. Undertaking research can be demanding in terms of resources, and opting for an excessively large sample size may prove unfeasible or impose significant financial strain. A sample that is too large can also be costly and time-consuming to collect and analyse. However, a larger sample size generally leads to more reliable results, as it reduces the margin of error and increases the likelihood of detecting true differences or relationships within the data. By increasing the size of the sample, researchers are able to identify more subtle effects or distinctions, resulting in enhanced accuracy when estimating population parameters (Lakens, 2022). This aspect holds particular significance in the realm of quantitative research, as it necessitates accurate calculations and universally applicable findings as the utmost priority. In addition, the careful selection of a suitable sample size aids in the efficient management of resource restrictions. For this reason, the goal of the study is to collect data from a minimum of 500 samples in order to circumvent the issue of a restricted sample size.

Using systematic random sampling design from the population at 95% confidence level and 5% confidence interval, a sample size of 384 was desired. In this study, we obtained a sample of 393 above the desired level.

- **Sampling unit:** The sample unit is the customer of the diagnostic centre who has availed of diagnostic services from any of the centres and he/she is in a position to respond. Here the customer may be the patient himself or his/her attendant in case of a minor and dependent person. Further, considering the unique nature of the industry, we anticipated that all the chosen customers would not be able to share the data with us, therefore, the size of the sample taken was larger initially. For this purpose, we studied the customer database for at least five months and undertook judgment sampling. Only those customers who fit into the following three categories were taken into consideration:

i. Repeat customers are those customers who have received at least three diagnostic services in the last three months;
ii. High-value customers, for our study, were those whose bill was more than Rs. 10,000;
iii. High-volume customers were those who have got at least three diagnostic tests in one go, but the bill amount is less than Rs. 10,000 (Banasiewicz, 2004; Cui et al., 2015; Stangl et al., 2017; Kim et al., 2004; Folkman & Norman, 2002).

The respondents were requested to give their opinion, based on five-point scales, concerning their degree of acceptance of various items to be included in the questionnaire framed keeping in view the objectives and hypotheses mentioned in the chapter.

- **Data analysis:** This section offers an elaborate explanation of the process of analysing data with the help of SPSS, which encompasses descriptive analysis such as mean, percentage, standard deviation etc., t-test, Cronbach's Alpha, factor analysis, Apriori algorithm for data mining etc.

The t-test is a statistical test used to determine if there is a significant difference between the means of two groups. It is commonly used when comparing the means of two independent groups or when comparing the mean of a sample to a known population mean. There are different types of t-tests, such as the independent samples t-test (for comparing means of two independent groups), paired samples t-test (for comparing means of two related groups), and one-sample t-test (for comparing the mean of a sample to a known value). The test calculates a t-statistic based on the sample data and compares it to a critical value from the t-distribution to determine if the difference between the means is statistically significant (Field, 2013; Kim, 2015).

Cronbach's Alpha, often referred to simply as Cronbach's alpha or coefficient alpha, is a measure of internal consistency reliability to assess the reliability of a scale or questionnaire. Cronbach's alpha ranges from 0 to 1, where higher values indicate greater internal consistency reliability. It measures the extent to which all items in a scale or questionnaire are measuring the same underlying construct. A Cronbach's alpha value of 0.70 or higher is generally considered acceptable for research purposes, although the specific threshold may vary depending on the context (Bland & Altman, 1997; Tavakol & Dennick, 2011).

Factor analysis is a statistical technique used to identify underlying factors or latent variables that explain the correlations among observed variables. It is commonly used to reduce the complexity of data and identify meaningful patterns. Factor analysis aims to group observed variables into clusters or factors based on their shared variance. These factors represent underlying constructs or dimensions that are not directly observable but are inferred from the patterns of correlations among the observed variables. Factor analysis results in factor loadings, which indicate the strength and direction of the relationship between each observed variable and each underlying factor. Researchers use factor analysis to explore the structure of data, confirm hypotheses about underlying constructs, and develop or refine measurement instruments such as scales or questionnaires (Hair et al., 2006; Costello & Osborne, 2019; Stevens, 2002).

- **Profile of the respondents:**

The profile of the respondents is given in Table 3.5.

Table 3.5: **Profile of the respondents**

Age of the Customer		
Age	Frequency	Percentage
Less than 25 Years	51	13.0
25 Years To 35 Years	109	27.7
35 Years To 45 Years	120	30.5
45 Years To 55 Years	56	14.3
More than 55 Years	57	14.5
Total	393	100
Gender of the Customer		
Gender	Frequency	Percentage
Male	180	45.8
Female	213	54.2
Total	393	100
Marital Status		
Marital Status	Frequency	Percentage
Married	332	84.5
Unmarried	61	15.5
Divorced	0	0
Widow/ Widower	0	0
Others	0	0
Total	393	100

Source: Author's compilation

- **Delimitations of the study:** Delimitations play a crucial role in a thesis as they establish the confines within which the research is conducted, ensuring clarity, focus, and feasibility. By setting boundaries, researchers can refine their research questions, objectives, and methods, enabling a more targeted and efficient investigation. This focused approach prevents the study from becoming overly broad or unwieldy, allowing for a detailed examination of specific aspects of interest. Additionally, delimitations enhance the confidence and clarity of the research by defining explicit parameters for both the researcher and the audience, ensuring the study's relevance, achievability, and practicality within its specified boundaries. Overall, delimitations provide researchers with a clear framework, guiding them through the complexities of their chosen topic and facilitating the generation of meaningful and impactful results. (Maxwell, 2012; Neuman, 2013).

The purpose of this study is to assess the customer experience, their perception towards the service quality and accountability of diagnostic centres. The analysis keeps a clear focus on diagnostic centres only, excluding other related areas of healthcare such as hospitals. This research is concentrated on customer experience, their perception of service quality and accountability in diagnostic centres, while excluding other types of experiences perception in hospitals. The factor analysis will prioritise key determinants identified in literature and empirical studies to investigate the factors influencing the customer experience and their perception of accountability in diagnostic centres. This excludes broader economic and regulatory factors that may influence experience and accountability in diagnostic centres.

The investigation will focus on current data and advancements within a specific timeframe (up to the present date), excluding historical analyses that exceed a certain duration. Future projections will only consider extrapolations based on current data and trends, rather than extensive speculation about long-term technological advancements or regulatory changes. Although the study uses a representative sample of population in India to ensure that the findings are relevant to the defined geographical area, the research's findings and conclusions may be universally applicable beyond the given geographical area under consideration.

3.4 Chapter Summary

This chapter outlined the approach that was utilized to address the research question and meet the goals of the study. There were four parts to the chapter. Initially, the research approach and data collection philosophy served as the foundation for establishing the framework for the research design employed in this study. This context prepared the audience for a discussion of the study's implementation of the research design. Second, the theoretical framework outlined in earlier chapters was used to generate research construct measures. The sampling strategy and the process used to choose the study participants were then covered. A discussion of the data analysis processes concludes the chapter.

Chapter 4

Analysis & Interpretation

Customers of diagnostic centres in Guwahati, Assam, India, were the subjects of this study to determine their experiences, perceptions of the centres' service quality, and accountability. Besides, the study was also done to find out the experiences of the customers on the basis of their complaints filed on the registered complaints portal. It is to be noted that complaints are the result of negative customer experiences and therefore, reflects the sentiment of the customers accordingly. This chapter covers the findings of the study in four sections. Firstly, the findings of the data mining applied on the customers complaints is extracted to find out the negative customer experiences of the customers. Secondly, the study attempts to find out the level of customers experiences and the factors them. Thirdly, the study reports the findings on service quality of the customers of diagnostic centres and finally, the customers perception of accountability is reported.

4.1 Customers Experiences on the Basis of their Complaints

To find common words and association rules, the complaint text and title were examined independently. This strategy was chosen since the complaint text's main points are frequently captured in the title. The ensuing subsections address the conclusions drawn from the study of the complaint text and the title.

4.1.1 Analysis of Title of the Complaints

The complaint titles were analyzed to identify frequent terms and association rules. Table 1 presents a list of single terms with their corresponding support, calculated using a minimum support threshold of 0.02 (Dietrich, 2015). This means that terms appearing in more than 2% of the complaints were selected for analysis. The frequency of words in Table 4.1 indicates that approximately 15.8% of complaints were related to reports, highlighting a potential area for improvement in customer experience. Notably, 14.7% of complaints were marked as resolved, suggesting a positive aspect of customer experience. Additionally, 15% of complaints concerned poor service quality, while 7.3% addressed staff behavior. Interestingly, 3.2% of complaints were related to COVID vaccination, and the same percentage of complaints used the terms “misleading” and “negligence” to describe the experience.

***Table 4.1:* Words with a maximum frequency in the title of complaints**

Words	Support
report	0.157894736842105
Resolved	0.147368421052632
Service	0.147368421052632
Test	0.094736842105263
Staff	0.073684210526316
Behavior	0.73684210526316
COVID	0.031578947368421
Negligence	0.031578947368421
Vaccination	0.031578947368421
Misleading	0.031578947368421

Source: Author's compilation

After analyzing the most frequent words, a group of two words with maximum frequency were calculated and the result was tabulated in Table 4.2.

***Table 4.2:* Group of two words with a maximum frequency in the title of complaints**

Words	Support
('report', 'test')	0.063157894736842
('service', 'poor')	0.042105263157895
('jp', 'nagar')	0.031578947368421
('behavior', 'rude')	0.021052631578947
('certificate', 'vaccine')	0.021052631578947
('salt', 'lake')	0.021052631578947
('medical', 'negligence')	0.021052631578947
('staff', 'misleading')	0.021052631578947
('wrong', 'report')	0.021052631578947
('time', 'waiting')	0.021052631578947

Source: Author's compilation

The data from Table 4.2 indicates a significant portion of customers (6.3%) have experienced difficulties obtaining test reports. Additionally, 4.2% of complaints specifically mentioned poor service as the source of their dissatisfaction. Furthermore, 2.1% of complaints cited specific issues such as rude behavior, medical negligence, misleading staff, lengthy wait times, problems with vaccine certificates, and incorrect test reports as contributing factors to their negative experiences. The data further reveals that the JP Nagar clinic accounts for the majority of complaints (3.2%), followed by the Salt-lake clinic (2.1%).

A group of three words that occurred together in a complaint has been tabulated in Table 4.3. The minimum support used to calculate the frequency of the terms was 0.02 (Dietrich, 2015).

***Table 4.3:* Group of three words with a maximum frequency in the complaints**

Words	Support
('jp', 'nagar', 'resolved')	0.031578947368421
('received', 'test', 'report')	0.021052631578947
('service', 'worst', 'nagar')	0.021052631578947
('lake', 'salt', 'resolved')	0.021052631578947

Source: Author's compilation

Table 4.3 shows that 3.1 percent of complaints were related to JP Nagar clinic while 2.1 percent of the complaints were related to Salt Lake clinic and included the term resolved. 2.1 percent of total complaints indicated problems in receiving test reports.

Table 4.4 contains groups of four words that occur in a single complaint. The minimum support used to calculate the frequency of the terms was 0.02 (Dietrich, 2015).

***Table 4.4:* Group of four words with a maximum frequency in the complaints**

Words	Support
('exp', 'worst', 'jp', 'nagar')	0.021052631578947
('exp', 'jp', 'nagar', 'resolved')	0.021052631578947

Source: Author's compilation

Table 4.4 reflects that about 2.1 percent of the complaints termed their experience as the worst and these complaints were related to JP Nagar. The same number of complaints were also marked as resolved.

In Figure 4.1, a word cloud has been generated to visually represent the frequency of the different terms in the title of the complaints. In figure 4.1, the size of the words signifies the frequency of the terms. The more the frequency of the term, the larger the size.

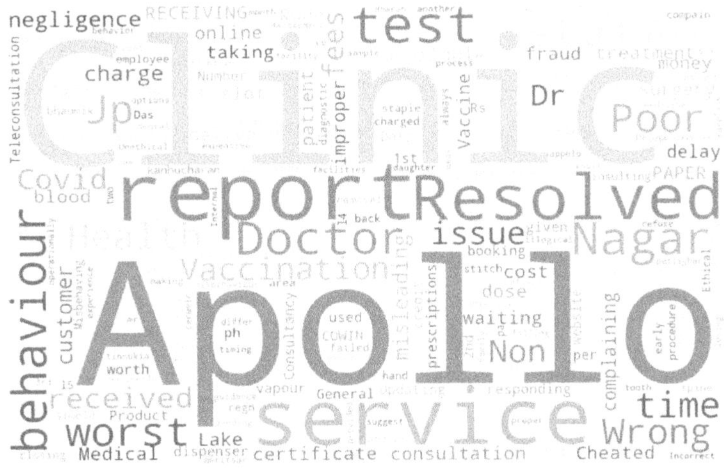

Source: Author's compilation

***Figure 4.1:* Word cloud generated from complaint title**

After analyzing the frequent terms, association rules were generated using association mining. The most significant rules are tabulated in Table 4.5. The minimum confidence level was specified at 0.7.

***Table 4.5:* Rules extracted from the title of the complaints**

Antecedent	Consequent	Confidence
Rude	Behavior	1
Vaccine	Certificate	1
Delay	Report	1
(jp, nagar)	Resolved	1
(salt, lake)	Resolved	1

Source: Author's compilation

The table 4.5 shows that whenever a delay is mentioned in a complaint, a report is also mentioned. Additionally, all complaints registered for the Salt Lake clinic and JP Nagar clinic have been resolved by the management. This suggests that there may be a link between delays and reports, and that the management is taking steps to address complaints.

Specifically, the table shows the following:

- "delay" and "report" have a confidence of 1.0, which means that whenever "delay" is mentioned, "report" is also mentioned.
- "Salt Lake clinic" and "resolved" have a confidence of 1.0, which means that all complaints registered for the Salt Lake clinic have been resolved.
- "JP Nagar clinic" and "resolved" have a confidence of 1.0, which means that all complaints registered for the JP Nagar clinic have been resolved.

An analysis of complaint texts revealed the most common terms and association rules.

***Table 4.6:* Words with a maximum frequency in the complaint texts**

Words	Support
Doctor	0.252631578947368
Test	0.273684210526316
Report	0.157894736842105
Service	0.126315789473684
Vaccine	0.042105263157895
Behavior	0.031578947368421
Behaviour	0.031578947368421
Unprofessional	0.031578947368421
Vaccination	0.031578947368421
Pathetic	0.031578947368421

Source: Author's compilation

Table 4.6 lists the single terms and their corresponding support values, with a minimum support of 0.02. Sorting the terms by support highlights the most frequently used terms. The data indicates that "test" (27.4%) and "report" (15.8%) were the most common terms, suggesting that 15.8% of complaints concerned test reports. "Service" (12.6%) was also prevalent, while "behavior" (3.2%), "unprofessional" (3.2%), and "pathetic" (3.2%) were used less frequently. This implies that at least 12.6% of complaints were related to poor service.

Table 4.7: **Group of two words with a maximum frequency in the complaint texts**

Words	Support
('report', 'test')	0.126315789473684
('checkup', 'health')	0.042105263157895
('experience', 'bad')	0.042105263157895
('appointment', 'refused')	0.021052631578947
('certificate', 'vaccine')	0.021052631578947
('first', 'vaccine')	0.021052631578947

Source: Author's compilation

The most frequent two-word terms in complaint texts were identified and tabulated in Table 4.7. The minimum support used to calculate term frequency was 0.02. Terms were sorted based on support for analysis. Table 4.7 shows that "test report" (12.6%) and "health checkup" (4.2%) were the most frequent two-word terms, indicating issues with these services. Additionally, "experience bad" (4.2%) and "appointment refused" (2.1%) were prevalent, suggesting problems with customer experience and appointment scheduling.

The most frequent three-word terms in complaint texts were identified and tabulated in Table 4.8. The combination of "report", "blood", and "test" appeared in 4.2% of complaints, with 1% specifically mentioning "wrong", highlighting challenges in obtaining blood test reports.

Table 4.8: **Group of three words with a maximum frequency in the complaint texts**

Words	Support
('report', 'test', 'doctor')	0.08421052631579
('report', 'blood', 'test')	0.042105263157895
('report', 'wrong', 'doctor')	0.031578947368421
('report', 'blood', 'wrong')	0.010526315789474

Source: Author's compilation

A word cloud in Figure 4.2 visualizes the frequency of terms in complaint texts. Larger words indicate higher frequency. Association rules generated from complaint texts provided no significant insights.

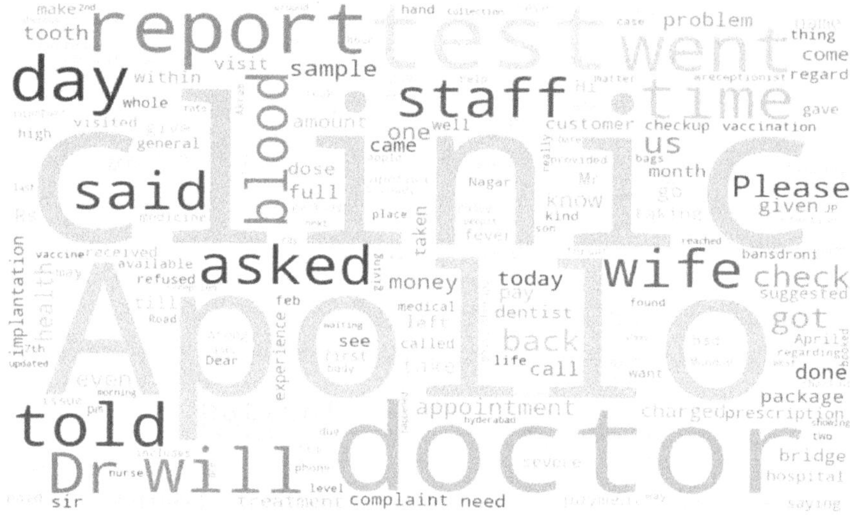

Source: Author's compilation

Figure 4.2: **Word cloud generated from complaint text**

4.1.2 Discussion

An analysis of complaints reveals that 12.6% of unfavorable experiences concern delays and errors in test reports, while 4.2% and 2.1% pertain to health checkups and COVID vaccinations, respectively. Delays in receiving test reports warrant serious attention. Such delays can cause patients undue suffering and exacerbate their ailments (Concannon et al., 2009). It is crucial to recognize that delays or errors in test reports can lead to misdiagnosis or inaccurate assessments during patient follow-ups. Consequently, procedures that combine error detection with a search for potential root causes are necessary to implement preventive and corrective measures. Customers also reported unfavorable experiences related to staff behavior, including "rude behavior" and "poor service" (4.2% each) and "medical negligence" (2.1%). Rudeness significantly impacts healthcare service delivery (Guo et al., 2022). Rude language and unpleasant behavior among diagnostic service providers jeopardize patient safety and the quality of care they receive (Flin, 2010). Frow & Payne (2007) found that customer satisfaction declines when services fall below expectations. Poor service leads to dissatisfaction, and unsatisfied customers are more likely to engage in negative word-of-mouth, switching providers, and complaining (Um & Lau, 2018). Poor provider attitudes can deter service utilization and foster low expectations and discriminatory behavior among healthcare providers (Devkota et al., 2017). Geographically, customers from JP Nagar and Salt Lake reported the highest frequency of unfavorable experiences. This study contributes to the existing body of knowledge in customer experience by examining unfavorable customer experiences in diagnostic centers, as reflected in customer complaints. The findings have managerial, policy, and theoretical implications.

4.2 Customer Experience in Diagnostic Centres

The overall experience of the customers in the diagnostic centres extracted on the basis of the response of the customers obtained through interview schedule is reported under the following headings:

4.2.1 The Scale and its Reliability

A reliability test of the scale was done and the Cronbach's Alpha coefficient was 0.908 for 28 items included in the research study. The high value of Cronbach's α indicates that the scale has a high reliability degree and there is a high correlation between the items and the items considered for the scale are actually measuring the latent variable (Field, 2009). The list of items considered in the scale along with their individual mean and standard deviation is depicted in Table 4.9.

Table 4.9: **Item Statistics**

Items	Mean	Std. Deviation
Giving intimation about the time of next check up	3.75	0.967
Not disclosing your personal information to others	3.64	1.020
Convenience of paying the requisite fees	3.63	0.928
Comfort with the way some personal information are asked	3.57	0.912
Getting help while filling up some forms	3.53	0.926
Comfort with the type of document sought	3.52	0.904
Explaining the process of doing diagnosis	3.51	0.904
Sitting facility	3.5	1.010
Clarification of doubts raised related to the diagnosis	3.49	0.784
Availability of the personnel at the diagnostic centre	3.49	0.870
Giving information about the time of delivery of report	3.49	0.937
Giving individual attention	3.48	0.881
To suggest the most suitable type of diagnosis	3.47	0.744
Ambience	3.44	0.913
To tell exactly when the services will be performed	3.43	0.781
To provide necessary help after diagnosis is done	3.42	0.955
Eager to solve problems at an earliest.	3.38	0.992
To suggest the most affordable way of diagnosis	3.37	0.824
To keep accurate records of previous reports	3.37	0.883
Waiting area	3.37	1.011
Willingness to provide service do not vary with each counter	3.34	0.819
Time required to get the report	3.29	0.935
Timely delivery of report	3.29	0.945
To keep you informed about any regulatory aspect	3.25	1.018
Parking facility	3.13	1.116
Help in getting insurance settlement	3.04	1.014
Online delivery of report	2.91	1.035
To give occasional gifts like diaries, calendars etc.	2.78	1.168

Source: Compiled from the interview schedule

4.2.2 Scale Construction and Interpretation

The scale consisted of 28 items and the maximum possible score in the scale computes to140 (28×5), whereas it is 28 (28×1) in case of minimum score. So, the difference or interval in the range comes to be 112 [140(max)-28(min)]. If 112 is divided by 5, a result of 22.4 is obtained. This 22.4 is added to28 (lowest possible score), then the range of 28-50.4 was achieved. In a similar way, rest of the intervals are obtained corresponding to many levels of customer experience. Singh (2012); Singh & Bhattacharjee (2019); Singh et al (2020); Singh et al (2021) have also adopted similar kind of scaling to measure latent variables. The interpretations obtained are given in table 4.10.

Table 4.10: **Customer Experience Score Interpretation**

Customer experience score interval	Interpretation
28.0-50.4	Very unfavourable experience
50.4-72.8	Unfavourable experience
72.8-95.2	Moderate experience
95.2-117.6	Favourable experience
117.6-140.0	Very favourable experience

Source: Authors' compilation

4.2.3 Overall Experience

Overall level of customer experience in diagnostic centre is depicted in Table 4.11.

Table 4.11: **Overall Experience**

Levels of customer experience	Frequency	Percent
Very unfavourable Experience	4	1.0
Unfavourable Experience	43	11.0
Neutral	126	32.0
Favourable experience	192	49.0
Very Favourable experience	28	7.0
Total	393	100.0
Mean		94.8800
Standard Deviation		308.693

Source: Author's compilation

It is observed above that the mean score is 94.88 which falls under moderate experience as explained in Table 4.10. Thus, it can be inferred that customers of the diagnostic centre have "moderately favourable experience".

4.2.4 Factor Analysis

Having understood the overall customer experience, the next question was to discover and then understand the factors or variables which affect the experience of customers in diagnostic centres.

To know the answer to this question, principal component analysis needs to be performed. The data suitability and sample size adequacy also need to be checked before proceeding for factor analysis. To achieve this, Keiser-Meyer-Olkin (KMO) and Bartlett tests (1954) are performed. This ensures that the results of factor analysis are reliable (Kaiser, 1974). The test values of KMO and Bartlett range from 0 to 1 (Field, 2009). According to Hutcheson & Sofroniou (1999) and Field (2009), the range and the sample adequacy along with the interpretation are - Below 0.5 is unacceptable, 05. to 0.7 is mediocre, 0.7 to 0.8 is good, 0.8 to 0.9 is great and above 0.9 is superb. The present research has the value of KMO to be above 0.5, thus it is adequate. Table 4.12 depicts the p-value to be 0.000 (>0.05). This can be a confirmation for the data appropriateness to proceed for factor analysis.

***Table 4.12:* KMO and Bartlett's Test**

Kaiser-Meyer-Olkin Measure of Sampling Adequacy.		.885
Bartlett's Test of Sphericity	Approx. Chi-Square	2025.404
	Df	378
	Sig.	.000

Source: Author's compilation

Table 4.13 depicts the extraction of the actual factors. The labelled "Rotation Sums of Squared Loadings" includes only such factors that meet the extraction method criteria. In the present research, the factors which have the Eigen value>1 are five in number. The "% of variance" column describes the overall variability. Here, 68.93% explanation of the total variability is done by the first 5 factors. This means that there are 5 components after the Principal Component Analysis.

***Table 4.13:* Total Variance Explained**

Component	Initial Eigenvalues			Rotation Sums of Squared Loadings		
	Total	% of Variance	Cumulative %	Total	% of Variance	Cumulative %
1	12.802	45.721	45.721	5.056	18.058	8.058
2	2.426	8.663	54.384	4.130	14.750	32.807
3	1.690	6.034	60.418	4.083	14.582	47.389
4	1.361	4.862	65.281	3.398	12.135	59.524
5	1.022	3.651	68.932	2.634	9.408	68.932
6	.871	3.109	72.041			
7	.841	3.002	75.043			
8	.723	2.584	77.627			
9	.681	2.432	80.059			
10	.572	2.041	82.100			
11	.550	1.964	84.064			
12	.492	1.756	85.820			
13	.438	1.565	87.385			
14	.422	1.507	88.892			

Component	Initial Eigenvalues			Rotation Sums of Squared Loadings		
	Total	% of Variance	Cumulative %	Total	% of Variance	Cumulative %
15	.376	1.343	90.234			
16	.354	1.264	91.499			
17	.317	1.132	92.631			
18	.309	1.103	93.733			
19	.274	.979	94.712			
20	.265	.948	95.660			
21	.226	.808	96.468			
22	.204	.727	97.195			
23	.180	.643	97.837			
24	.158	.563	98.400			
25	.154	.549	98.949			
26	.116	.416	99.365			
27	.108	.387	99.752			
28	.070	.248	100.000			

Source: Author's compilation

Table 4.14: **Rotated Component Matrix**[a]

	Component				
	1	2	3	4	5
Ambience	**.806**	.225	.188	.172	.119
Waiting area	**.791**	.097	.218	.138	.307
Sitting facility	**.733**	.069	.252	.112	.282
Willingness to provide service do not vary with each counter	**.667**	.390	.319	.193	-.030
Giving individual attention	**.637**	.302	.250	.174	.096
Parking facility	**.570**	.110	.256	.466	.148
To tell exactly when the services will be performed	**.552**	.550	.068	.165	.145
To keep accurate records of previous reports	**.537**	.253	.135	.351	.196
To keep you informed about any regulatory aspect	**.496**	.392	.224	.339	.198
Getting help while filling up some forms	.323	**.718**	.176	.120	.179
Comfort with the type of document sought	.247	**.708**	.237	.223	.316
Comfort with the way some personal information are asked	.102	**.700**	.239	.313	.297
To provide necessary help after diagnosis is done	.181	**.595**	.303	.409	.147
Giving Intimation about the time of next check up	.212	**.563**	.394	-.062	.343
Eager to solve problems at an earliest.	.445	**.485**	.230	.371	-.075
Clarification of doubts raised related to the diagnosis	.210	.123	**.798**	-.004	.209
Explaining the process of doing diagnosis	.178	.223	**.735**	.246	.053
To suggest the most suitable type of diagnosis	.205	.217	**.715**	.076	.066

	Component				
	1	2	3	4	5
To suggest the most affordable way of diagnosis	.232	.058	**.712**	.328	-.182
Not disclosing your personal information to others	.106	.422	**.587**	-.270	.146
Availability of the personnel at the diagnostic center	.377	.149	**.543**	.004	.338
Convenience of paying the requisite fees	.341	.446	**.495**	-.067	.409
To give occasional gifts like diaries, calendars etc.	.246	.090	.021	**.838**	-.051
Online delivery of report	.159	.139	.053	**.772**	.295
Help in getting insurance settlement	.233	.275	.054	**.696**	.308
Giving information about the time of delivery of report	.233	.367	-.015	.121	**.761**
Timely delivery of report	.251	.238	.284	.343	**.677**
Time required to get the report	.281	.260	.152	.387	**.585**
Extraction Method: Principal Component Analysis. Rotation Method: Varimax with Kaiser Normalization.					
a. Rotation converged in 8 iterations.					

Source: Author's compilation

Table 4.14 shows the rotated factor loadings. It represents the weight of the variables for each component along with the explanation of the correlation between the components and the variables. This also identifies the items that can be grouped under one group and for which one common nomenclature is to be used and thus, total factors can be reduced. At last, the final components located are presented in Table 4.15.

Table 4.15: **Items Included**

Components		**Name of the Components**
1	• Ambience • Waiting area • Sitting facility • Willingness to provide service do not vary with each counter • Giving individual attention • Parking facility • Tell exactly when the services will be performed • Keep accurate records of previous reports • Keep you informed about regulatory aspect	Requisite infrastructure
2	• Getting help while filling up some forms • Comfort with the type of document sought • Comfort with the way some personal information are asked • Provide necessary help after diagnosis is done • Giving intimation about the time of next check-up • Eager to solve problems at an earliest	Comfort of dealing

Components		Name of the Components
3	• Clarification of doubts raised related to the diagnosis • Explaining the process of diagnosis • Suggest the most suitable type of diagnosis • Suggest the most affordable way of diagnosis • Not disclosing your personal information to others • Availability of the personnel at the diagnostic centre • Convenience of paying the requisite fees	Empathetic treatment
4	• Give occasional gifts like diaries, calendars, etc. • Online delivery of report • Help in getting insurance settlement	Ancillary services
5	• Giving information about the time of delivery of report • Timely delivery of report • Time required to get the report	Accessibility and availability

Source: Author's compilation

4.2.5 Discussion

The study showed moderate level of customer experience among the customers of the diagnostic centres. It also unearths the top items contributing to favorable customer experience identified as 'giving intimation about the time of next check-up', 'not disclosing personal information to others', and 'convenience of paying the requisite fee'. Worlu (2016) explains the behavior of the consumers in a health facility. The consumers are mostly unclear regarding their safety and well-being leading to fear. Therefore, health seekers are very anxious to have their privacy protected (Fox et al., 2000). Patients look for supportive and helping behaviour which includes being caring and attentive (Naidu, 2009). Tucker (2002) found that the degree, to which the patient is heard, provided with understandable and relevant information, given enough time during consultation are significant. The top most reasons responsible for receiving unfavorable customer experience are 'help in getting insurance settlement', 'online delivery of report', and 'receiving occasional gifts like diaries, calendars, etc.'. From the consumers' perspective, it is very crucial to have clarity on some aspects of the service or product during the point of sale (Jain et al., 2014). Related to this is the role of insurers because they administer and carve a business based on the benefits plans to the customers who are patients (Vargas et al, 2012). Table 4.8 gives us the 5 top most factors with mean value 3.5 and above impacting experience. It would be useful for the managers to focus on the areas of concern.

Finally, our research has also helped us to discover the factors which affect the experience of customers in diagnostic centres which are broadly classified as 'requisite infrastructure', 'comfort of dealing', 'empathetic treatment', 'Ancillary services', 'Accessibility and availability' (Table 4.15). This categorization would further make the task of experience management convenient and effective. Johnston & Kong (2011) emphasized that among the factors such as value for money, reliability, problem solving etc., reliability is the most important. The emotional aspects include assurance, trust and care. The access to diagnostic facilities relates to its availability at the time of requirement and the meetings between patient and physician (Turner & Pol, 1995). Organizations need to gain novel insights from analysis of such experiences along with prior managers' knowledge (Lam et al, 2017).

4.3 Customers' Perception of Service Quality of Diagnostic Centres

Service quality is evaluated by patients based on their perceptions of the services they have received. To assess the quality of these services, patients/customers compare their perceptions with their initial expectations. The Diagnostic Centres' Customers' Perception of Service Quality extracted on the basis of the response of the customers obtained through interview schedule is reported under the following headings.

4.3.1 Reliability of the Questionnaire

Table 4.16: **Reliability Statistics**

Dimension of Customer Perception/Expectation	Cronbach's Alpha		No. of Items
	Perception	Expectation	
Tangibility	0.733	.657	4
Reliability	0.713	.607	5
Responsiveness	0.679	.676	4
Assurance	0.703	.545	4
Empathy	0.614	.900	5

Source: Author's compilation

The internal consistency of the scale was assessed using Cronbach's alpha. While all scales exceeded the traditionally recommended threshold of 0.70 for reliability (Nunnally, 1978), a few values fell slightly below this benchmark. Given the first-time use of the scale in a diagnostic centre setting, a Cronbach's alpha of 0.60 or higher was considered acceptable in this context (Vaske et al., 2017).

4.3.2 Perception and Expectation Towards Tangibility of Diagnostic Centres

The item statistics of the first component of service quality named tangibility is presented in table 4.17.

It is evident from table 4.17 that up-to-date equipment in the clinic have been given perceived relatively more important by the customers whereas employees' dress is given relatively less importance to evaluate the overall tangibility of the diagnostic centre. So far as the expectation is concerned, up-to-date equipment in the clinic have been most expected feature of a diagnostic centre by the customers whereas appearance of physical facilities with the type of services is given relatively least expected.

Table 4.17: **Item Statistics**

Tangibility items	Perception		Expectation	
	Mean	**Std. Deviation**	**Mean**	**Std. Deviation**
Up-to-date equipment in the clinic	2.4097	1.47517	4.8499	.39169
Visually appealing physical facilities	2.3181	1.47188	4.8244	.41920
Very well dressed and neat appearance of employees	2.1730	1.45356	4.6896	.53483
The appearance of the physical facilities of the clinic is in keeping with the type of services provided	2.3969	1.48296	4.6209	.54984
Overall Mean	9.2977 12.796		18.9847	
Overall Std. Deviation		1.32086		

Source: Author's compilation

The interpretation table for tangibility, which was assessed using four items on a five-point Likert scale, is displayed in Table 4.18. On a scale of 1 to 5, the respondents were asked to rate the same after the variables were changed into statements. Here 1 represents 'Very unfavourable Perception of Tangibility and 5 represents 'Very Favourable Perception of Tangibility. For a scale consisting of 4-items, the maximum possible score was 20 (4*5) and minimum possible score is 4 (4*1), giving a difference of 16 (20-4). This difference (16) was divided by 5 to show the 5 perception-layers regarding Tangibility, giving a value of (3.2). Therefore, the 1st level of perception score with respect to tangibility is between 4 and 7.2 (4+3.2), and is interpreted as 'Very unfavourable perception of tangibility'. Similarly, other levels are calculated, as shown in Table 4.18, to show the different levels of customer's perception (Agarwal & Singh, 2023).

Table 4.18: **Interpretation Table to interpret perception and expectation score of Tangibility and its present status**

Perception/ Expectation score interval	Interpretation	Perception (P)		Expectation (E)	
		Scores	**Percentage**	**Scores**	**Percentage**
4-7.2	Very unfavourable perception /expectation of Tangibility	177	45.0	0	0
7.2-10.4	Unfavourable perception /expectation of Tangibility	95	24.2	0	0
10.4-13.6	Moderate perception /expectation of Tangibility	86	21.9	3	.8
13.6-16.8	Favourable perception /expectation of Tangibility	35	8.9	14	3.6
16.8-20	Very Favourable perception /expectation of Tangibility	0	0	376	95.7
	Total	393	100	393	100

Source: Author's compilation

Since overall mean (9.29) shown in table 4.17 falls in the category of 'Unfavourable perception of tangibility' it can be said that overall perception of customers towards tangibility is unfavourable. Majority (i.e., 177+95= 272) of the customers of diagnostic centres have unfavourable perception about the tangibles dimension of service quality. However, the mean score for expectation as reflected in table 4.17 is 18.98, which falls under very high expectation of tangibility. Thus, it can be interpreted that customers of the diagnostic centres expect the tangibles to be very good.

4.3.3 *Perception and Expectation Towards Reliability of Diagnostic Centres*

Table 4.19: **Item Statistics**

	Perception		**Expectation**	
Reliability items	**Mean**	**Std. Deviation**	**Mean**	**Std. Deviation**
Clinic's commitment to meet deadlines	2.6489	1.41740	4.5878	.62926
Clinic's support for customer issues	2.5776	1.44445	4.6361	.55551
Dependability of the clinic	2.3130	1.34250	4.5700	.65917
On-time services	2.1018	1.40328	4.7201	.49798
Accurate record-keeping	2.2850	1.45868	4.7303	.49849
Overall Mean	11.9262 3.46810		23.2443	
Overall Std. Deviation		1.77464		

Source: Author's compilation

Table 4.19 shows that customers perceive the reliability of the clinics as relatively higher with respect to the factors like "commitment to meet deadlines" and "support for customer issues." Customers perceive relatively lower reliability of diagnostic centres with respect to the factor like "On-time services". Whereas, 'accurate record keeping' and 'on-time services' are the most expected features of reliability of diagnostic centre.

As explained in Table 4.18, an interpretation table is made considering the five items taken for measuring customers' perception regarding reliability and it is presented in Table 4.20. The mean score is 11.9. It falls under low level of perceived reliability. Thus, it can be interpreted that customers of the diagnostic centres perceive that the services of the clinics are not very reliable. On the other hand, the mean score for expected reliability is 23.24. It falls under very highly expected reliability. Thus, it can be interpreted that customers expect the diagnostic centres to be very highly reliable.

Table 4.20: **Interpretation Table to interpret perception and expectation Score of Reliability and its present status**

Perception/ Expectation score interval	Interpretation	Perception (P)		Expectation (E)	
		Scores	Percentage	Scores	Percentage
5-9	Very low level of perceived/ expected reliability	99	25.2	0	0
9-13	Low level of perceived/ expected reliability	130	33.1	0	0
13-17	Moderately perceived/ expected reliability	116	29.5	3	.8
17-21	Highly perceived/expected reliability	48	12.2	52	13.2
21-25	Very highly perceived/ expected reliability	0	0	338	86.0
	Total	393	100	393	100

Source: Author's compilation

4.3.4 Perception and Expectation Towards Responsiveness of Diagnostic Centres

Table 4.21: **Item Statistics**

	Perception		Expectation	
Responsiveness items	**Mean**	**Std. Deviation**	**Mean**	**Std. Deviation**
Clinic lacks service time specificity.	2.2087	.59524	2.3537	.83885
Slow service from clinic staff.	2.1501	.47419	2.1934	.51335
Inconsistent willingness of clinic staff to assist.	2.2417	.52981	2.1552	.46162
Clinic staff overwhelmed with customer requests.	2.5191	.58490	2.4478	.57406
Overall Mean	9.1196		9.1501	
Overall Std. Deviation	1.54967		1.69644	

Source: Author's compilation

Table 4.21 shows that customers perceive the responsiveness of the clinics as relatively higher with respect to the factor like "Clinic staff overwhelmed with customer requests" Customers perceive relatively lower responsiveness of diagnostic centres with respect to the factor like "Slow service from clinic staff". On the expectation size, the customers expect the clinic to be highly responsive with respect to the factor like "Clinic staff overwhelmed with customer requests" followed by "Clinic lacks service time specificity" whereas willingness of staff to assist customer is least expected by the customers.

The interpretation table to interpret the perception and expectation score of responsiveness along with its present status is given in table 4.22.

Table 4.22: **Interpretation Table to interpret perception and expectation score of responsiveness and its present status**

		Perception (P)		Expectation (E)	
Perception/ Expectation score interval	**Interpretation**	**Scores**	**Percentage**	**Scores**	**Percentage**
4-7.2	Very low level of perceived/ expected responsiveness	14	3.6	10	2.5
7.2-10.4	Low level of perceived/ expected responsiveness	326	83.0	324	82.4
10.4-13.6	Moderately perceived/ expected responsiveness	46	11.7	48	12.2
13.6-16.8	Highly perceived/ expected responsiveness	7	1.8	9	2.3
16.8-20	Very highly perceived/ expected responsiveness	0	0	2	.5
	Total	393	100	393	100

Source: Author's compilation

By looking at the scale statistic in Table 4.21, the mean score is 9.11. It falls under low level of perceived responsiveness. Thus, it can be interpreted that customers of the diagnostic centres perceive that the services of the clinics are not very responsive, however, the mean value for the expected responsiveness is 9.15. It falls under low level of expected responsiveness. Thus, it can be interpreted that customers do not expect the diagnostic centres to be very responsive.

4.3.5 Perception and Expectation Towards Assurance of Diagnostic Centres

Table 4.23: **Item Statistics**

	Perception		Expectation	
Assurance items	**Mean**	**Std. Deviation**	**Mean**	**Std. Deviation**
Confident in clinic staff.	1.8295	1.29321	4.7303	.57011
Confident in clinic transactions.	2.3053	1.46677	4.5802	.55725
Politeness of the staff	2.5980	1.47468	4.6845	.55068
Clinic staff receives ample support.	2.1298	1.41275	4.6463	.72463
Overall Mean	8.8626		18.6412	
Overall Std. Deviation	2.82237		1.56526	

Source: Author's compilation

Looking at table 4.23, it is evident that politeness of the employees has been given relatively more importance by the customers whereas confidence in the clinic staff is given relatively less importance, as perceived by the customers. On the contrary, confidence in the clinic staff is the most expected feature of assurance dimension of service quality of diagnostic centres followed by politeness of the staff.

Interpretation table of perception and expectation score of the assurance dimension of service quality of diagnostic centres along with its present status is given in table 4.24.

Table 4.24: **Interpretation table to interpret perception and expectation score of assurance and its present status**

Perception/Expectation (P/E) score	Interpretation	Perception (P)		Expectation (E)	
		Scores	Percentage	Scores	Percentage
4-7.2	Very low level of perceived/ expected assurance	199	50.6	0	**0**
7.2-10.4	Low level of perceived/expected assurance	121	30.8	1	.3
10.4-13.6	Moderately perceived/expected assurance	47	12.0	7	1.8
13.6-16.8	Highly perceived/expected assurance	26	6.6	24	6.1
16.8-20	Very highly perceived/expected assurance	0	0	361	91.9
	Total	393	100	393	100

Source: Author's compilation

By looking at the scale statistic in Table 4.23, the mean score is 8.86. It falls under low level of perceived assurance. Thus, it can be interpreted that customers of the diagnostic centres are not very assured about their services. Contrary to that the mean score of expected assurance is 18.64. It falls under very highly expected assurance. Thus, it can be interpreted that customers expect the services of the diagnostic centres to be very highly assured.

It is evident from table 4.25 that convenient operating hour followed by customer centric approach have been given perceived as relatively more important by the customers whereas individual attention is given perceived relatively less important. On the expectation size also, the similar trend is visible.

4.3.6 *Perception and Expectation Towards Empathy of Diagnostic Centres*

Table 4.25: **Item Statistics**

Empathy items	Perception		Expectation	
	Mean	Std. Deviation	Mean	Std. Deviation
Lacks personalized customer focus.	2.2366	.57364	2.2163	.55008
Clinic staff lacks personalized customer care.	2.2468	.53227	2.2036	.55263
Clinic staff unaware of customer needs.	2.4580	.56595	2.2672	.55546

	Perception		Expectation	
Empathy items	**Mean**	**Std. Deviation**	**Mean**	**Std. Deviation**
Clinic lacks customer-centric approach.	2.5623	.56857	2.4148	.61734
Convenient operating hours for all.	3.7684	.54849	2.5445	.64971
Overall Mean	13.2721		11.6463	
Overall Std. Deviation	1.75100		2.46808	

Source: Author's compilation

The interpretation table of perception and expectation score of empathy dimension of service quality of diagnostic centre along with its present status is given in table 4.26.

Table 4.26: **Interpretation table to interpret perception and expectation score of empathy and its present status**

		Perception (P)		Expectation (E)	
Perception/ Expectation (P/E) score	**Interpretation**	**Scores**	**Percentage**	**Scores**	**Percentage**
5-9	Very low level of perceived/ expected empathy	6	1.5	5	1.3
9-13	Low level of perceived/ expected empathy	138	35.1	283	72.0
13-17	Moderately perceived/ expected empathy	237	60.3	96	24.4
17-21	Highly perceived/ expected empathy	12	3.1	7	1.8
21-25	Very highly perceived/ expected empathy	0	0	2	0.5
	Total	393	100	393	100

Source: Author's compilation

By looking at the scale statistic in Table 4.26, the mean perception score of is 13.27 falls under moderately perceived empathy. Thus, it can be interpreted that customers of the diagnostic centres have moderate perception of empathy. On the other hand, the mean expectation score is 11.6. It falls under low level of expected empathy. Thus, it can be interpreted that customers of the diagnostic centres expect the services of the clinics to be less empathetic.

4.3.7 Overall Analysis

The overall expectation of the customers of diagnostic centres with respect to service quality is given in table 4.27.

Table 4.27: **Overall expectation of service quality of diagnostic services**

	Frequency	Percent
Very low expectation of service quality of diagnostic centres	0	0
Low expectation of service quality of diagnostic centres	0	0
Moderate expectation of service quality of diagnostic centres	11	2.8
High expectation of service quality of diagnostic centres	381	96.9
Very high expectation of service quality of diagnostic centres	1	0.3
Total	393	100

Source: Author's compilation

The overall perception of the customers of diagnostic centres with respect to service quality is given in table 4.28.

Table 4.28: **Overall perception of service quality of diagnostic centres**

	Frequency	Percent
Very unfavourable perception of service quality of diagnostic centres	8	2.0
Unfavourable perception of service quality of diagnostic centres	304	77.4
Moderate perception of service quality of diagnostic centres	73	18.6
Favourable perception of service quality of diagnostic centres	8	2.0
Very Favourable perception of service quality of diagnostic centres	0	0
Total	393	100

Source: Author's compilation

Seeing table 4.27 and 4.28, it is concluded that overall expectation of the customers of the diagnostic centres is high (96.9) but their perception of the same service is very unfavourable (77.4).

To test the significance of difference of mean values of perception and expectation of respective dimension of service quality, t-test is performed. The result of the t-test is given in the table 4.29.

Table 4.29: **Paired Samples Statistics**

	Mean	Std. Deviation	P-E	t	Sig. (2-tailed)
Tangibility_P	9.2977	3.57720	-9.68702	-46.352	.000
Tangibility_E	18.9847	1.32086			
Reliability_P	11.9262	3.46810	-11.31807	-53.654	.000
Reliability_E	23.2443	1.77464			
Responsiveness_P	9.1196	1.54967	-0.03053	-0.330	0.741
Responsiveness_E	9.1501	1.69644			
Assurance_P	8.8626	2.82237	-9.77863	-53.609	.000
Assurance_E	18.6412	1.56526			
Empathy_P	13.2723	1.75100	1.62595	12.899	.000
Empathy_E	11.6463	2.46808			

Source: Author's compilation

Table 4.29 represents the paired t-test results of different factors between Perception score vs Expectation score. It has been observed that there is no significant difference between perception vs expectation with respect to the factor responsiveness (p-value being 0.74). However, for other pairs it is found to be significant as the p-value is 0.000 (i.e. < 0.05). The table shows that only for empathy, the perception is higher than the expectation which means customers are satisfied with the empathy dimension of service quality (+ 1.63). However, for other three dimensions, the perception scores are lower than the expectation scores which says that there is a service quality gap with regard to dimensions such as tangibility, reliability and assurance.

***Table 4.30:* Results on hypotheses**

Expectation	Perception	Gap	Hypotheses (accepted/Rejected)
Tangibility	Tangibility	Negative	Rejected
Reliability	Reliability	Negative	Rejected
Responsiveness	Responsiveness	No Gap	Accepted
Assurance	Assurance	Negative	Rejected
Empathy	Empathy	Positive	Rejected

Source: Author's compilation

Hence the hypothesis that there is no significant difference between expectation and perception of customers of diagnostic centres with respect to various dimensions of service quality is rejected with respect to tangibility, reliability, assurance and empathy dimensions.

4.3.8 Discussion

The discrepancies between expectation and perception in respect of Tangibility, Reliability, and Assurance show that customers' actual experiences did not satisfy their initial expectations. These aspects can be improved to better align client perceptions with their expectations. For responsiveness, customers' opinions of timely service and employee willingness closely matched their expectations, as seen by the tiny disparity. However, for empathy, while there was a positive gap, showing that expectations were surpassed, this dimension highlighted the facilities' strength in providing personalized care. In general, service quality was lower than the expectations of the customers in the studied diagnostic centers.

Identifying the gaps in service quality dimensions and employing proper policies will lead to an improvement and patient's satisfaction. Healthcare diagnostic centers should focus on updating facilities, enhancing consistency, and creating trust to bridge the gaps in tangibility, reliability, and assurance (Zeithaml et al., 1990). Maintaining the existing positive alignment between perceptions and expectations will be critical for maintaining customer satisfaction in terms of responsiveness and empathy.

Overall, the study offers useful insights into specific aspects of service quality where healthcare diagnostic centers may improve and align consumer views with their expectations. Healthcare diagnostic facilities can improve client satisfaction, loyalty, and reputation by correcting gaps in tangibility, reliability, and assurance while keeping the current favorable view in responsiveness and empathy. A customer-centric strategy, combined with investments in technology and personnel training, has the potential to significantly improve service quality and overall performance for these centers (Sheth et al., 2023).

4.4 Accountability

The result of customers perception of accountability of diagnostic centres extracted on the basis of the response of the customers obtained through interview schedule is reported under the following headings:

4.4.1 The Scale and its Reliability

The scale consists of the items collected on a five-point Likert scale, with a response of strongly disagree receiving a score of 1, signifying a very low degree of accountability, and strongly agree receiving a score of 5, signifying a very high level of accountability. Only response number 14 is intended to be contradictory. When item-total correlation was applied to the aforementioned items, it was discovered that items No. 6, No. 9, and No. 14 had item-total correlation values that were less than 0.2. This indicates that these things do not correlate well with the overall score and may be eliminated. Hence, 11 items in all were used for analysis. The reliability of the data was tested using Cronbach's Alpha. Using Cronbach's alpha, it was determined whether the scale designed to gauge the degree of perceived accountability of diagnostic facilities was reliable. Cronbach's alpha has a value of 0.638. If a scale is created and used for the first time, a Cronbach's alpha of higher than 0.60 is said to be a solid indicator of its reliability (Nunnaly 1978). As a result, it can be concluded from the current study that the scale is reliable and capable of measuring the latent variable known as accountability.

Table 4.31 lists, in descending order, the item statistics of the 11 items that were taken into consideration for the scale to assess customers perception of accountability.

Table 4.31: **Item Statistics**

	Mean	Std. Deviation
Getting test reports delivered on time.	4.6310	.71339
Perception regarding the authenticity and reliability of the reports generated by the diagnostic center.	4.5674	.61125
Getting timely reminders for tests to be done afterward.	4.5623	.69386
Getting justifiable reasons for the actions performed by the diagnostic center for any particular test.	4.2137	.74239
Possession of requisite qualifications by the lab technicians to perform the tasks.	4.0509	.87625
Possession of requisite qualifications by the pathologist to perform the tasks.	4.0483	.88940
In case of any error, taking responsibility by the diagnostic center for its action.	3.8779	.82706
Following the requisite protocols for all diagnoses and tests.	3.6616	.75591
In case of any error, run the test, again free of cost.	3.4784	.89509
In case of any error, conduct a thorough inquiry to find out the cause behind the error.	3.3842	.84059
Using the latest technology prevalent in the relevant healthcare diagnostic industry for all the diagnoses and tests.	3.2010	.66455

Source: Author's compilation

Table 4.31 shows the factors contributing the most toward the favorable customers' perception of accountability of diagnostic centres. The top three factors having the maximum impact on overall favourable customers' perception of accountability are 'getting the reports on time by the customers' (4.63), 'agree to the authenticity and reliability of the reports' (4.57), and 'getting timely reminders for the next tests' (4.56). The factors least important in framing the customers' overall level of perception of accountability are, 'in case of any error, running the test, again free of cost' (3.4784); 'conducting a thorough inquiry to find out the cause behind the error' (3.3842); 'using the latest technology prevalent in the relevant healthcare diagnostic industry for all the diagnoses and tests' (3.2010).

4.4.2 Status of Customers Perception of Accountability of Diagnostic Centres

The scale used to gauge customers' perceptions of responsibility had 11 components. The maximum possible score computes to be 55 (11x5), and the lowest score is 11 (11x1). Thus, the difference or range interval is 44 [55 (max)-11(min)]. When 44 is divided by 5, the answer is 8.8. The range of 11-19.8 is reached by adding this 8.8 to the lowest possible score of 11. Similarly, the rest of the intervals correspond to many customers' perception levels. The interpretations of customers' perception of accountability score and overall accountability are given in Table 4.32.

Table 4.32: **Customers' perception of accountability score and overall accountability**

Customer perception score interval	**Interpretation**	**Frequency**	**Percent**
11.0-19.8	Very Low level of perception of accountability	0	0
19.8-28.6	Low level of perception of accountability	0	0
28.6-37.4	Moderate level of perception of accountability	19	4.83
37.4-46.2	High level of perception of accountability	268	68.20
46.2-55.0	Very High level of perception of accountability	106	26.97
Total		393	100
Overall mean			43.68
Standard Deviation			3.985

Source: Author's compilation

Figure 4.3: Presents the different levels of customers perception accountability.

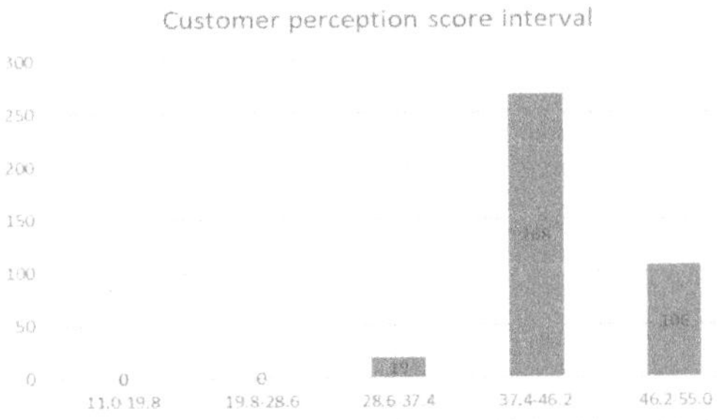

Source: Author's compilation

Figure 4.3: **Graphical representation of customers perception of accountability of diagnostic services**

It has been noted that the overall mean score is 43.68 which lies in the interval 37.4-46.2, representing a "high level of accountability". Hence, it may be concluded that the users of the diagnostic centres in Guwahati have a favourable perception of the accountability of diagnostic centres.

4.4.3 Factor Analysis

Checking the appropriateness of the sample used for the study is the first step in performing factor analysis. The Kaiser-Meyer-Olkin (KMO) measure of sample adequacy and Bartlett's test were applied to the 393 replies in order to evaluate the data's applicability gathered from the samples. The KMO and Bartlett's test of sphericity determines whether there is an overlap between the variables and whether they can be reduced to a handful of parameters. The identical goal of both tests is to confirm that the original variables can be used effectively in the factor analysis. The result of the above test is presented in Table 4.33.

Table 4.33: **KMO and Bartlett's Test**

Kaiser-Meyer-Olkin Measure of Sampling Adequacy.		.568
Bartlett's Test of Sphericity	Approx. Chi-Square	1617.384
	Df	55
	Sig.	0.000

Source: Author's compilation

The Kaiser-Meyer Olkin Measure (KMO) of Sampling Adequacy and Bartlett's Test of Sphericity (significant level of p.05) should be used to examine whether the given dataset has patterned relationships and whether the data set is appropriate for exploratory factor analysis (Yong & Pearce, 2013). The sample is sufficient as the result of KMO was 0.57, which is greater than 0.5. It is noteworthy since Bartlett's Test of Sphericity significance value is less than.05. Table 4.34 presents the Eigenvalues and explanation of total variance.

Table 4.34: **Total Variance Explained**

Component	**Initial Eigenvalues**			**Rotation Sums of Squared Loadings**		
	Total	**% of Variance**	**Cumulative %**	**Total**	**% of Variance**	**Cumulative %**
1	2.657	24.152	24.152	2.350	21.360	21.360
2	2.014	18.307	42.459	2.070	18.817	40.177
3	1.661	15.096	57.555	1.711	15.557	55.734
4	1.454	13.222	70.776	1.655	15.042	**70.776**
5	.783	7.117	77.894			
6	.672	6.113	84.007			
7	.589	5.355	89.362			

Component	Initial Eigenvalues			Rotation Sums of Squared Loadings		
	Total	% of Variance	Cumulative %	Total	% of Variance	Cumulative %
8	.405	3.679	93.042			
9	.383	3.484	96.526			
10	.299	2.723	99.248			
11	.083	.752	100.000			
Extraction Method: Principal Component Analysis.						

Source: Author's compilation

The real factors' extraction is shown in Table 4.35. Only those components that satisfy the extraction method requirements are included in the section titled "Rotation Sums of Squared Loadings." There are four components in the current study with Eigen values greater than 1. The overall variability is described in the "% of variation" column. Here, the first 4 components account for 70.78% of the total variability. As a result, the Principal Component Analysis has produced 4 components. The principal component analysis is used to identify the variables that are most closely related to each component or which of these values are of significant size. Finding the variables with low correlation to the component is made easier using this technique. Larger correlations are bolded in Table 4.35's Rotated Component Matrix, which displays the results.

Table 4.35: **Rotated Component Matrix**[a]

	Component			
	1	2	3	4
Possession of requisite qualifications by the pathologist to perform the tasks.	**0.943**	0.081	-0.046	0.063
Possession of requisite qualifications by the lab technicians to perform the tasks.	**0.924**	0.033	0.005	-0.037
In case of any error, taking responsibility by the diagnostic centre for its actions.	**0.633**	0.068	-0.145	0.532
Getting test reports delivered on time.	-0.046	**0.838**	-0.034	0.072
Perception regarding the authenticity and reliability of the reports generated by the diagnostic centre.	0.222	**0.751**	0.146	-0.005
Getting timely reminders for tests to be done afterwards.	-0.204	**0.692**	-0.096	0.313
Getting justifiable reasons for the actions performed by the diagnostic centre for any particular test.	0.253	**0.55**	0.057	-0.27
Following the requisite protocols for all diagnoses and tests.	0.051	0.072	**0.865**	-0.105
Using the latest technology prevalent in the relevant healthcare diagnostic industry for all the diagnoses and tests.	-0.129	-0.026	**0.849**	0.146

	Component			
	1	2	3	4
In case of any error, run the test, again free of cost.	0.155	0.033	-0.085	**0.861**
In case of any error, conduct a thorough enquiry to find out the cause behind the error.	-0.077	0.054	0.419	**0.645**
Extraction Method: Principal Component Analysis.				
Rotation Method: Varimax with Kaiser Normalization.				
a. Rotation converged in 5 iterations.				

Source: Author's compilation

The rotational factor loadings are shown in Table 4.35. It illustrates the importance of the variables for each component and explains how the variables and components are related. Also, it highlights the things that can be put into groups and for which a single common nomenclature should be used, allowing for the reduction of the total number of elements. The final components discovered are shown in Table 4.36 as a last step.

Table 4.36: **Results of factor analysis**

Component	**Items included**	**Name of Component**
1	• Possession of requisite qualifications by the pathologist to perform the tasks. • Possession of requisite qualifications by the lab technicians to perform the tasks. • In case of any error, taking responsibility by the diagnostic centre for its actions.	Competency
2	• Getting test reports delivered on time. • Perception regarding the authenticity and reliability of the reports generated by the diagnostic centre. • Getting timely reminders for tests to be done afterwards. • Getting justifiable reasons for the actions performed by the diagnostic centre for any particular test.	Responsiveness
3	• Following the requisite protocols for all diagnoses and tests. • Using the latest technology prevalent in the relevant healthcare diagnostic industry for all the diagnoses and tests.	Compliance with the protocol
4	• In case of any error, run the test, again free of cost. • In case of any error, conduct a thorough enquiry to find out the cause behind the error.	Problem-solving approach

Source: Author's compilation

4.4.4 Discussion

The above analysis addresses two research questions. RQ7 attempts to measure the level of customers' perception of accountability of healthcare diagnostic service providers. It was found that the general level of customer perception with respect to accountability of diagnostic centres is of high level. The items such as 'getting test reports delivered on time', 'perception regarding the authenticity and reliability of the reports generated by the diagnostic center', and 'getting timely reminders for tests to be done afterward', have a substantial impact on creating the public's favourable view of accountability. RQ8 was to find out the factors influencing the perception of accountability of healthcare diagnostic service customers. The study identifies four factors that have an impact on the perception of customers with respect to the accountability of diagnostic service providers. These are Competency, Responsiveness, Compliance with protocol, and Problem-solving approach. Meaningful accountability only results when all four factors are effective.

Veres, Locklear, and Sims (1990) founds that the main components of competency are the information, skills, and personal qualities that employees must have in order to execute their jobs well. All of these characteristics are anticipated to have an impact on how accountable a healthcare company is. Keel (2006) states that competency is described as a set of behaviours that includes skills, knowledge, talents, and personal characteristics that, when combined, are essential for successfully completing work tasks. Improvements in competency lead to advancements in accountability in the same direction (Bakalikwira et al., 2017). Since the delivery of quality care service to patients depends on employees, organizational efficiencies, and treatment processes, hospital systems should encompass the competences to handle the needs of both the provider and patients (Lee et al. 2012; Lee 2018).

Diane et al. (2012) states that managerial abilities offer a solid foundation for increased accountability. This also leads to an improvement in professional accountability as propounded by Romzek & Dubnick, (2018). The second factor influencing the perception of customers with respect to the accountability of diagnostic service providers is responsiveness. Responsiveness entails responding readily and sympathetically to some request (Thomas, 1998). The healthcare industry is a complicated, safety-critical field where technology mistakes can directly injure patients (Sittig & Singh, 2015). A crucial component of accountability is the existence of complaint and response systems that allow interested parties to voice complaints and claim harm and obtain responses (Blagescu, et al., 2005). Responsiveness ensures an increase in the customers' perception of legal and professional accountability (Romzek & Dubnick, 2018). The third factor influencing the perception of accountability is compliance with protocols. Compliance with protocol means adherence to laws, guidelines, regulations, and specifications applicable to healthcare diagnostic business processes. Compliance is crucial, particularly in the heavily regulated, risky healthcare sector. The ultimate purpose of compliance in the healthcare business is to offer patients with safe, high-quality care by adhering to industry norms and regulations. The fourth factor is a problem-solving approach which means identifying and analysing the patients' needs and providing the best solution to solve the problem which further necessitates effective communication and teamwork. Mukinda et al., (2020) discovered that the absence of communication was perceived as a roadblock to accountability, which had an impact on the standard of care and fostered a culture of finger-pointing and shifting of blame. Proper communication facilitates solving the problem. Problem-solving approach increases the customers' perception of political and professional accountability as suggested by Romzek & Dubnick (2018) and ensures the promotion of public health and community benefit as suggested by Emanuel & Emanuel, (1996).

Hence, the four core dimensions that make an organization more accountable to its stakeholders can be explained and aligned with the accountability theories mentioned in chapter 1 of the thesis.

Knowledge, skills, abilities, personal traits, and other "worker-based" factors make up the first component of **competency** as supported by Vance et al., (2013). The second-factor **responsiveness** is responding as quickly as possible to a situation. Alertness, approachability, awareness, impartiality. Frink et al., (2008) supported this in the accountability theory proposed by them. The next factor is **compliance with the protocol** which means adherence to laws, guidelines, regulations, and specifications applicable to healthcare diagnostic business processes as supported by Blagescu et al., (2005). Finally, the **problem-solving approach** addresses the need to identify and analyse the patients' needs and provide the best solution to solve the problem as suggested by Vance et al., (2015) in the accountability theory proposed by them.

Thus, it is seen that the four factors impacting the perception of customers with respect to the accountability of diagnostic service providers as identified in this study are also linked with the existing theories of accountability.

The dimensions are interconnected and have various effects on one another. A diagnostic centre must incorporate these aspects into its practices, rules, and decision-making at all levels and phases in order to be held accountable.

4.5 Chapter Summary

This chapter provides a thorough examination of the data, their analysis and interpretation. This stage of research is critical for any research project as it is the point at which all of the conceptualization has been tested on actual data. The researcher presented the respondents' demographic profile and checked the reliability of each construct. Following that, the researcher conducted objective wise data analysis using various tools and techniques as appropriate. The researcher discussed the findings and discussion based on the results of the analysis. The results conforming the first objective highlighted the unfavorable experiences of customers in diagnostic centres which is reflected in customers' complaints about delay in test reports, wrong test reports, rude behavior of the staff, poor service, and medical negligence. Customers of the diagnostic centers had a somewhat positive degree of customer experience, according to the study's second objective. It also discovered the factors which affect the experience of customers in diagnostic centres which are broadly classified as 'requisite infrastructure', 'comfort of dealing', 'empathetic treatment', 'Ancillary services', 'Accessibility and availability'. The analysis on the third objective concluded that the overall expectation of the customers of the diagnostic centres was higher than their perception of the same service indicating that there was a service quality gap with regard to dimensions such as tangibility, reliability and assurance. Ultimately, the fourth objective was also accomplished, and it was discovered that customers generally have a positive opinion of diagnostic centers' accountability. According to the study, there are four variables that influence how consumers view the accountability of diagnostic service providers. Competency, responsiveness, protocol compliance, and problem-solving methodology are these. Lastly, the aim of the study was to thoroughly examine how customers perceive and experience service quality and accountability, which would further offer recommendations for improvement.

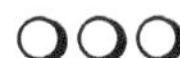

Chapter 5

Overall Conclusion, Academic Contributions, Implications, Limitations and Scope of Future Work

This study is undertaken with an objective to unearth some of the hidden aspects of diagnostic centres which is largely ignored till date. There have been a lot of study on hospitals and healthcare however, diagnostic services industry is largely ignored. This study attempts to bridge this gap. The overall conclusive findings of this study are presented in section 5.1.

5.1 Overall Conclusion

The first objective of the study was to identify the items affecting customers' experience from their complaints using data mining technique. Corollary of this objective was in the form of a research questions RQ1 which goes as "RQ1: What are the negative customer experiences that lead to customer complaints?" Research indicates that the majority of unfavourable encounters with diagnostic centres are related to errors and delays in test result processing, health examinations, and COVID-19 immunizations, in that order. Additionally, clients expressed negative encounters with employees' conduct, including "rude behavior", "poor service" and "medical negligence". The empirical results of this study offer innovation to the body of research by emphasizing the robust relationship between customer experiences in diagnostic centers and complaints from customers. It also demonstrates how the use of data mining tools has changed traditional CRM practices in healthcare industry, enabling good outcomes and evidence-based assessment. Extensive data on customer experiences will promote research-based support for the developing world's growing customer experience sector (Borishade et al., 2018). This research led to the development of the suggested framework shown in Figure 5.1.

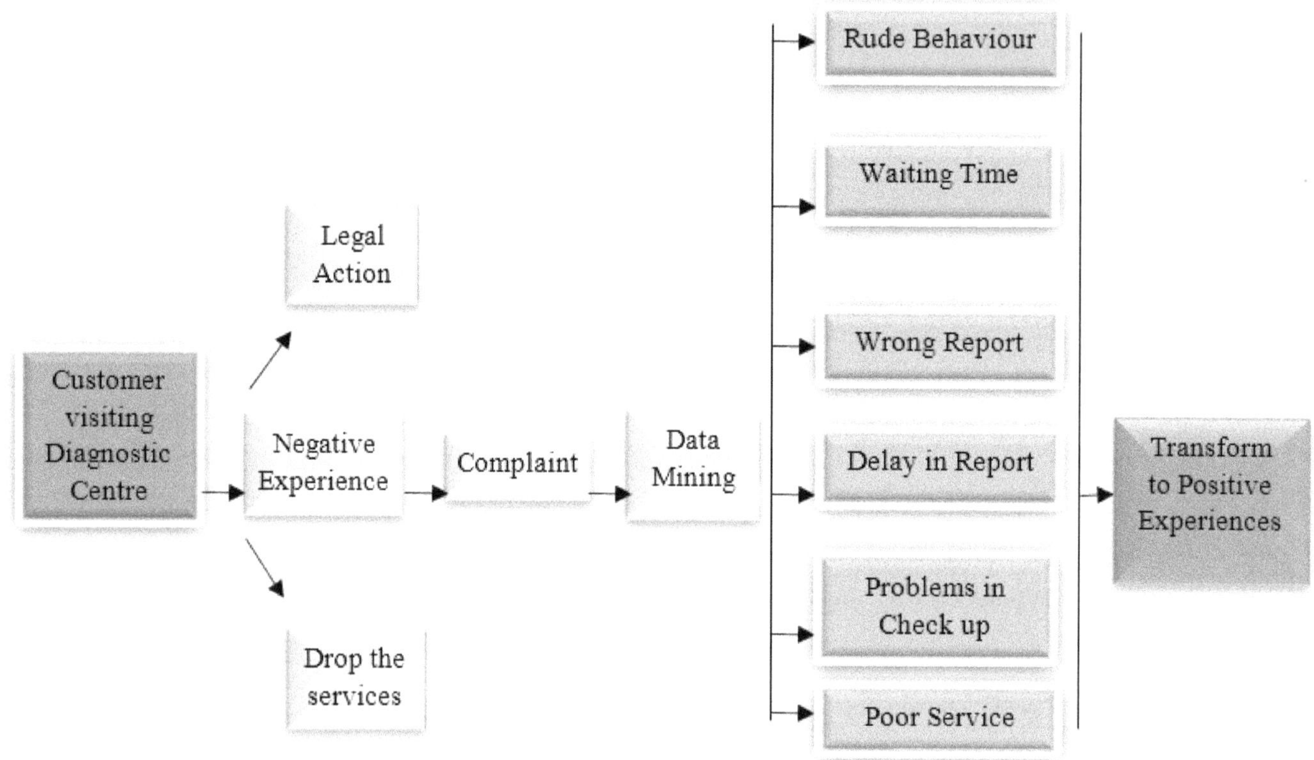

Source: Author's compilation

Figure 5.1: **Proposed model of Customer Experience in diagnostic centers**

The study's overall findings strengthen the reliability of the customer experience scale in diagnostic center environments and advance our theoretical knowledge of the experience concept in healthcare, and offer marketers of diagnostic centers insightful information. Positive or unpleasant experiences are possible for customers who visit diagnostic facilities. Three things can happen as a result of bad experiences: one can file more complaints, file a lawsuit, or find another supplier. Analysis of customer complaints is necessary for classification and further research. By doing this, the number of customers who switch to other diagnostic facilities may be decreased. According to Jeffrey et al., (2014), just 30% of companies use customer experience data to pinpoint problems and strengthen their position in the market. Instead of contacting the business directly, disgruntled customers frequently switch providers and complain about their bad experiences (Gal & Doron, 2007). Finally, diagnostic centers should begin to view any negative customer experiences as service issues and work to turn them into positive ones. This is because, although most customer experiences may not fall under the legal category and customers may not pursue legal action, it is still crucial for marketers to gain the loyalty of their clients and stay competitive in today's market. Bolton et al., (2018) emphasize the difficulties in fusing the digital, physical, and social domains to provide better customer experiences.

Second objective of the study was to investigate the experience of the customers of the diagnostics centre concerning various dimensions of services. Two research questions were attempted to be answered to fulfil this objective. RQ 2 goes as "RQ2: What is the overall level of customer experience in diagnostic centres?" and RQ3 is "RQ3: What are the factors influencing customer experience?" It was found that customers of the diagnostic centre have moderately favourable experience with the services of the diagnostic centres. To answer RQ2, it was found that the elements that impact patients' experiences at diagnostic centres are 'requisite infrastructure', 'comfort of dealing', 'empathetic treatment', 'ancillary services', 'accessibility and availability'. This research examines comparable pathways and presents conclusions in the form of elements to be used for enhanced customer experience, building on the work of Baranova (2017), which examined the customer's relationship with the company in light of the services offered. In order to precisely and thoroughly evaluate the client experience across the board for medical and health services, as well as in other domains of customer experience research, future research can make use of these particular results (Garg et al., 2010). By applying the scientific technique to a wider range of enterprises, further research in the field of customer experience can be conducted.

The third objective was to investigate how clients see different aspects of the diagnostic centre's service quality. The following research questions were framed to fulfil this objective:

- RQ4: What is the overall level of customer expectation with respect to service quality of diagnostic centres?
- RQ5: What is the overall level of customer perception with respect to service quality of their diagnostic centres?
- RQ6: Is there any gap between expectation and perception of customers of diagnostic centres with respect to various dimensions of service quality?

One hypothesis was also tested to fulfil this objective which is given hereinunder:

- $H0_1$: There is no significant difference between expectation and perception of customers of diagnostic centres with respect to various dimensions of service quality.

In response to RQ4, it was found that the customers of the diagnostic centres expect the tangibles to be of very high level. Customers expect the diagnostic services to be of very highly reliable. Assurance dimension of the service quality is also expected to be of very high level, however, with respect to the responsiveness and empathy, they expect it to be of low level.

In response to RQ5, it was found that the customers of diagnostic centres have unfavourable perception about the tangibles dimension of service quality, they have low level of perceived reliability about the diagnostic services. They have very low level of perceived assurance about the service of diagnostic centres. Their perception towards the tangibility dimension of service quality is also very unfavourable, however, with respect to that of the empathy, it is of moderate level.

So far as RQ6 was concerned, it was found that only for empathy, the perception is higher than the expectation which means customers are satisfied with the empathy dimension of service quality. There is no significant gap between the perception and expectation scores of responsiveness. However, for other three dimensions, the perception scores are lower than the expectation scores which says that there is a service quality gap with regard to dimensions such as tangibility, reliability and assurance.

H_{01} was tested and it was found that there is no significant difference between perception vs expectation with respect to the factor responsiveness ($p>0.05$). However, for other pairs such as tangibility, reliability, assurance and empathy, the hypothesis is rejected meaning thereby, the differences are significant ($p<0.05$).

Finally, the SERVQUAL tool proved to be reliable and valid in assessing service quality in diagnostic health-care setting. The analysis of data demonstrates the importance of delivering high-quality services in assuring happy patient experiences and improved healthcare outcomes. The findings emphasize the multifaceted nature of service quality, with dimensions such as reliability, responsiveness, tangibles, assurance, and empathy playing critical roles. The viewpoints and experiences of patients have been investigated, offering insight into the significance of patient satisfaction, preferences, and expectations. Understanding these insights allows healthcare facilities to modify their strategy to better serve their target population and increase overall customer satisfaction. Addressing service quality gaps can result in a competitive advantage in the healthcare industry. Despite this, researchers and stakeholders should be mindful of the study's limitations and perform additional research to validate and expand on the findings.

Finally, the fourth objective was to study the customer's perception of accountability of the service providers. Connected to this objective was the RQ7 and RQ8 which is given below:

- RQ7: What is the overall level of customer's perception of accountability of diagnostic centres?
- RQ8: What are the factors influencing the customer's perception of accountability of diagnostic centres?

In response to RQ7, it was discovered that the diagnostic centres' customers had a positive opinion of their accountability. In response to RQ8, it was discovered that four variables influence how customers see diagnostic centres' accountability. Competency, responsiveness, protocol compliance, and problem-solving methodology are these. In order for a diagnostic centre to be considered responsible by its clients, it must be responsive, follow procedures, hire qualified staff, and be capable of handling clients' issues. Figure 5.2 provides an explanation of this as the model to investigate how customers perceive diagnostic centres' accountability.

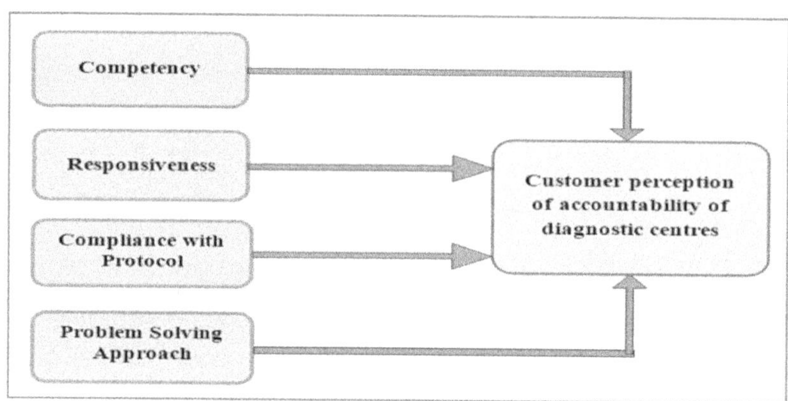

Source: Author's compilation

Figure 5.2: **Theoretical model showing customers' perception of accountability in diagnostic centres**

This expanded awareness of accountability permits the capacity to recognize and foster concepts that will promote accountability and raise the standard for diagnostic services. There are various ways to be accountable, and there are many different ways to fulfil it. This study demonstrates the significance of accountability in diagnostic centres for delivering excellent customer service (Singh et al., 2022). Therefore, an essential part of any complex healthcare system is the implicit promise given by healthcare organizations and professionals to patients to act with competence, take appropriate precautions, and offer recovery (Habli et al., 2020). Rather than being seen as an issue that has to be fixed, accountability ought to be seen as a continuous process that may be enhanced. The relationships that exist between healthcare providers, patients, and institutions are the foundation of healthcare. Beyond control and punishment, healthcare delivery services should be underpinned by their commitment to foster improved learning and improvement (Kerkvoorden et al., 2022). Ultimately, the questions surrounding the objectives of health sector accountability programs need to be revisited. Besides the efficacy and calibre of the health services, one may consider the citizenship of the users and the work ethics of the providers.

5.2 Academic Contributions

The academic contributions of this study are given under the following points:

1. Customer's complaint can be processed to understand the negative experiences of the customers which can be taken seriously by the diagnostic centres to be removed that can result into customer satisfaction. It is to be understood by the organisations that complaints are essentially the result of negative experiences of the customers. Therefore, there should be some mechanism, model or algorithm to process these complaints and help the users to identify the broad negative customer experiences. This study provides one such algorithm;
2. This study evaluated customer experience, customer impression of service quality, and service accountability in a methodical and thorough manner. While many academics have focused on applications in other industries to improve and evaluate customer experiences and service quality, diagnostic centres have not been the focus of their efforts. The goal of this study is to assist diagnostic centres in better understanding and utilizing the characteristics of client experiences, service quality, and accountability in order to increase income. The goal was to conduct a comprehensive analysis of consumer views and experiences in order to generate more guidelines for enhancement;
3. The research work makes significant contributions and broadens the body of knowledge in this field. It has determined what elements affect consumers' experiences and opinions about diagnostic centres;
4. This study offers up new avenues for empirical research in different geographical areas, which will subsequently help highly sensitive service industries like health care maintain and grow their consumer base. Drosos et al., (2015) address how data provided by patients aid in qualitative improvement. An effective analysis of this data is required to find trends and insights;

5. This study has provided consistent and reliable results arising out of empirical analysis to be followed in upcoming researches in the area of customer experience, service quality and accountability of diagnostic centres;
6. A first-of-its-kind model has been created to assess the quality of service, customer experience, and accountability for the diagnostic centre's services.;
7. This study contributes to the existing literature by framing a measurement scale for customer experience and view of accountability in diagnostic centres;
8. The study provides the empirical evidence that the five dimensions-SERVQUAL scale proved to be reliable and valid instrument for measuring and analysing health-care diagnostic service quality.
9. The established dimensions of service quality in healthcare diagnostic centres, such as reliability, responsiveness, tangibles, assurance, and empathy, give a theoretical framework for understanding the important components that contribute to service quality in the context of diagnostic centres. These characteristics can be used to lay the groundwork for future research and theoretical advancements in the field of healthcare service quality. This study adds to the conversation and sheds light on the broader implications and considerations surrounding service quality in the context of diagnostic services (Davis, 2019);
10. In addition to emphasizing the most and least significant aspects impacting the customers' sense of accountability in a diagnostic centre, this study provides four dimensions—a first for this kind of research—to measure accountability in diagnostic centres;
11. A significant academic contribution of this work is the creation of a theoretical model to explain customer experience and diagnostic centre accountability.

5.3 Managerial Implication

The managerial implications of the study are given hereinafter:

1. Using data mining techniques, the study could identify important aspects like rudeness, carelessness when delivering results, delayed reports, problems with checkups, and poor service. Certain issues are related to employee behavior and can be addressed by appropriate recruitment, training, and other measures; other aspects are related to flaws in the infrastructure. Analyzing and turning these complaints into satisfying client experiences ought to be the aim;
2. Improving the customer experience in diagnostic centres necessitates a multidimensional strategy that includes customer-centricity, decision-making based on data, and complaint handling. Howarth et al., (2015) emphasize complaints' relevance in customer retention (Platt, 2010) and argue that complaints should be seen as opportunities for development. According to Satish & Yusof (2017), data-driven decision-making requires employee training to use consumer data efficiently (Mela & Moorman, 2018);
3. According to Kirkland and Hyman (2021), personnel should be encouraged to Put people skills first and address patient complaints as a means of preventing communication breakdowns by framing patient experiences as customer service issues. Corrective action can be implemented

in accordance with the areas of improvement, which are clearly visible from the online ratings and feedback (Agarwal et al., 2024). In order to evaluate progress and make informed decisions going forward, Holmlund et al., (2020) advocate using key indicators to quantify the effectiveness of customer experience enhancement efforts;

4. Taking a customer-centric stance and giving their demands and perspectives top priority, can significantly enhance customer satisfaction. Schiavone et al., (2020), Ponsignon et al., (2018), and Lee (2017) highlight the benefits of this approach, suggesting that healthcare organizations can create more personalized, responsive, and effective service experiences;
5. Managers should adopt a management strategy that sees complaint resolution as a tactic for customer retention and organizational learning in place of the limiting legal paradigm for addressing complaints. A robust complaint handling system built on understanding, empathy, action, and honesty can benefit all parties involved (Howarth et al., 2015). Griffey & Bohan (2008) and Nikitha et al., (2020) advocate for a proactive approach to complaint management, encouraging diagnostic center managers to embrace new data analytics technologies to investigate unfavorable customer experiences and identify root causes;
6. The ever-growing array of technology demands flexibility and an openness to investigating novel methods of providing services (Foroudi et al., 2018). Managers should utilize natural language processing and sentiment analysis techniques to transform unstructured patient experience reports into actionable metrics of healthcare performance, particularly in diagnostic services. Greaves et al., (2013) offer a technique for deriving insightful information from patient input.
7. Healthcare marketers should place a high premium on hiring frontline employees with strong interpersonal and technical abilities in order to provide a remarkable customer service experience (Kashif et al., 2016).
8. Singh et al. (2021) recommends using the roster technique to handle COVID vaccination-related problems, streamlining the vaccination process, reducing wait times, and minimizing patient inconvenience. Diagnostic center managers should implement a reliable and 24/7 customer experience solution to provide decision-makers with continuous access to actionable insights. Holmlund et al., (2020) emphasize the importance of real-time data availability for informed decision-making;
9. Providing a remarkable and outstanding experience gives an organization a competitive advantage (Pine and Gilmore, 1999). There is an opportunity to convert the negative experience of the customers into positive ones adding to the overall productivity (Berry et al., 2002). So, it's quite obvious for the marketers to think in the direction of improving the customer experience (Garg et al., 2010) in this ever-increasing competition. So, identifying these factors and implementing them is very crucial in transforming the healthcare delivery system (Tajpour et al., 2020);
10. Giving clients gifts on occasion is one way that managers can contribute to an unpleasant experience, but they also need to realize that doing so would increase organizational costs, which upper management must carefully consider before making a final decision;

11. The process of enhancing quality can make use of technology and customer experience management (Tarmizi et al., 2021). A diagnostic centre should use modern technology to keep the data base of the customers and keep the customers informed about its various procedures and considering the fact that people are gradually becoming familiar with the use of Smart Phone and other devices (Singh et al., 2020), this step will help in building better understanding among the customers about the diagnostic centre;
12. Diagnostic center administrators can benchmark their actions against those of their rivals in the health-care market and enhance their operational performance by utilizing the SERVQUAL model;
13. Addressing tangibility, reliability, and assurance gaps can lead to increased customer satisfaction and loyalty. The research also emphasizes the significance of empathy in creating excellent customer experiences;
14. Diagnostic centres can improve their understanding of service quality and work toward implementing measures that promote patient satisfaction, safety, and overall healthcare excellence (Al-Ababneh, 2018) by applying the findings of this study;
15. The factors such as timely delivery of reports and reminders, authenticity and reliability of reports, being responsive by giving justifiable reasons, and requirement of requisite qualifications are essential to build favourable perception of accountability of diagnostic centres. The managers must work on these factors;
16. The formation of a "just culture" of accountability, learning, and growth is necessary at the individual and organizational levels (Hilber et al., 2016);
17. Training curricula ought to prioritize the empowerment of healthcare professionals (Rao et al., 2018). Training should include the specific ways that laws and regulations apply to the work that diagnostic service professionals do as well as the issues that they really encounter on a daily basis with healthcare compliance. Through this type of focused, practical training, staff members can learn how to apply policies and procedures to particular situations and what to look out for;
18. Healthcare practitioners and managers require supportive organizational frameworks since time management is especially sensitive in this sector. To fulfil their responsibilities and provide patient care, all healthcare professionals should make use of effective time management strategies (Kidak, 2011, Erolu & Zgür, 2016);
19. For the purpose of doing their jobs and providing patient care, all employees in the healthcare industry should understand how to manage their time well. It is imperative that they possess the ability to articulate the goals and objectives necessary to fulfil their specific professional duties. Worker self-management skills and increased personal accountability are also required due to changing trends and the makeup of the workforce (Dose & Klimoski, 1995);
20. There needs to be a high level of commitment from the board and top management levels inside the company for the dimensions to be implemented successfully and for businesses and stakeholders to benefit equitably from accountability (Blagescu, et al., 2005).

5.4 Policy Implications

The policy implications of this study are presented under the following points:

1. This study suggests a multifaceted strategy to close the practitioner-academic divide in handling patient complaints in the healthcare industry. Customer relationship managers should use interpersonal techniques to address complaints without placing blame, and customer complaints should be seen as service failures rather than legal issues (Olsson, 2016; Kirkland & Hyman, 2021). Diagnostic centers should place a higher priority on creating and implementing an efficient complaint management system and making sure their clients have a positive experience;
2. To manage performance, examine complaints, and address complainants, the management model should be enhanced by a centralized regulatory framework (Vogus & McClelland, 2016; Park et al., 2016). This approach could enhance diagnostic service quality and empower patients to file lawsuits without waiting for an internal grievance process, expanding legal remedies for medical negligence;
3. Governments should monitor hospital services and the health industry's situation to ensure that individuals are regarded as citizens first and as customers second (Agarwal et al., 2023);
4. It is obvious that policymakers must rethink and formulate health financing reforms to specifically target the socioeconomic population (Wasike, 2020). However, in this health care sector, the financial problem of expenditure is an issue for the households working in informal sector without insurance (Gumber & Kulkarni, 2000; Roy et al., 2017). This is important because one of the sources of generating unfavourable customer experience is the lack of help extended in getting insurance claim;
5. Lawmakers should also create legislation requiring any entity planning to operate a diagnostic center to ensure that it has a minimum amount of physical facilities (Singh & Choudhury, 2017);
6. To ensure that patients receive the degree of medical care they seek, service quality must be enhanced (Rooney & Van Ostenberg, 1999). To improve service quality, policymakers' efforts should be directed at continuous quality improvement, interprofessional collaboration, patient education, effective communication, patient safety measures, and the incorporation of technology;
7. Policies, standards, and regulatory frameworks should support and reward diagnostic centres for providing high-quality services. (Gounaris, 2021);
8. Accountability for the performance of service providers and the health administration is primarily enforced by the Ministry of Health and other government agencies. Depending on the level of non-compliance, government regulatory authorities may issue fines (Boydell et al., 2019);
9. A diagnostic centre should have a written statement of its promises to the client groups it serves regarding the services and/or plans that are being or will be offered to them. The document or charter may include protocols to be followed, the justification to be given for

some procedures, timely delivery of test reports, and reminders of the next tests which would further enhance the responsiveness and problem-solving approach of the diagnostic centre (Brinkerhoff, 2004);

10. There should be a proper mechanism to ensure transparency regarding the qualifications and competencies of the pathologists and the lab technicians. The patient or the customer should be educated beforehand about the procedure and actions to be performed by the diagnostic centre for a particular test;
11. Strong policies and procedures must be easily accessible and available, as this helps to guarantee compliance (Olsen, 2014). It is important for the policies to be explicit about the expectations, since this promotes organizational accountability;
12. In order to create a health system that is more responsive to health requirements, a Grievance Redressal System via help desks, call centres, and web portals should be in place. A partnership that focuses on learning and improvement rather than control and sanctions may be established, even if accountability is a crucial component in improving the governance and management of healthcare organizations and systems (Denis, 2014).

5.5 Limitations of the Study

Any academic work is not free from limitations. This study is also subject to certain limitations. This is given under the following paragraphs:

1. The negative customer experiences were extracted by processing the customer complaints registered on a specific consumer complaints portal. In order to generalise the findings, more such portals should be considered;
2. The algorithm used in the study to process customer complaints is Apriori algorithm. It is an old algorithm and there are many advanced algorithms developed by the scholars to analyse such data;
3. The research looked at the problem from the Indian users' perspective. The conditions, circumstances and situations are different in different countries and hence the findings cannot be generalised for the whole world;
4. The data was derived from a specific sample, which may not be representative of the total population. More study with larger and more diverse samples is required to reach more solid results and generalizations;
5. The limitations of sample survey are also applicable to this study. Every sampling design has certain limitations and despite the best efforts taken by the researcher to eliminate bias from the study, bias may be there in the data;
6. The present research primarily examines diagnostic center service quality in a broad sense, with little emphasis on individual diagnostic modalities (e.g., radiology, pathology, cardiology);
7. The study does not attempt to study impact of demographic variables, socio-economic variables on the customers experience, service quality and accountability;
8. Inter-relationship between the variables have not been studied.

5.6 Scope of Future Research

1. This study proposes future research directions and provides examples of fruitful ways to explore the connection between customer complaints and customer experience. The Apriori algorithm, while an established tool, has limitations compared to newer data mining techniques;
2. The study was carried out in the years 2021 and 2022, during and after the COVID-19 pandemic, hence its conclusions might not apply to other circumstances. To confirm these results, data collection from consumers under typical circumstances should be a focus of future research;
3. To gain a deeper understanding of the customer experience that connects offline consumer complaints and experiences with service delivery, descriptive research is required;
4. To generalize the results, more cross-sectional and longitudinal research are needed (Singh et al., 2022);
5. In this study, only patients who visit diagnostic centres in Guwahati are included. Thus, there is a chance to conduct in-depth research throughout the whole of Assam (Singh et al., 2022);
6. This study offers insightful information about patients' perceptions, but senior administrators of the clinic as well as the opinions of the pathologists, radiologists, lab technicians, and nurses can also be regarded as potentially rich information sources;
7. An exploratory study can be carried out to find out how people view accountability and service quality in connection to different demographic parameters and to determine how patient satisfaction is impacted by perceptions of accountability and service quality;
8. Various factors, varying in significance, impact customer experiences, service quality, and accountability. To ascertain this correlation, researchers can utilize the relationship between the parameters and social network analysis (SNA) (Kajol et al., 2020; Singh et al., 2021);
9. Future studies may examine conducting a comparison analysis that looks into the experiences and perceptions of various customer types and locations;
10. Factor moderation and mediation have not been included in the study. Future studies are encouraged by the authors to examine the mediation and moderating effects of other parameters;
11. Finally, a variety of associated subjects, such as the function of service providers or other stakeholders, might be investigated;
12. Future research can look into the complexities and particular problems of providing high-quality diagnostic services in specific diagnostic specialties.

5.7 Conclusion

The client experience, service quality, and accountability of the services rendered by diagnostic centers have all been thoroughly and methodically evaluated in this study. Numerous academics have focused on applications in various industries to improve and evaluate consumer experiences, but not in diagnostic centers. The goal of this study was to assist diagnostic centres in better understanding and using client experiences and perceptions to increase revenue. In order to further provide suggestions for improvement, a detailed analysis of customer experience and perception about service quality and accountability was intended. The research project makes significant contributions and broadens the body of knowledge in this field. It has determined what aspects of diagnostic centres affect customers' perceptions and experiences. Second, it has produced dependable and consistent empirical analysis results that will be used in future studies on customer experience, service quality, and accountability. Thirdly, models have been developed to measure the customer experience, service quality, and accountability with respect to the services of a diagnostic centre, which is first of its kind.

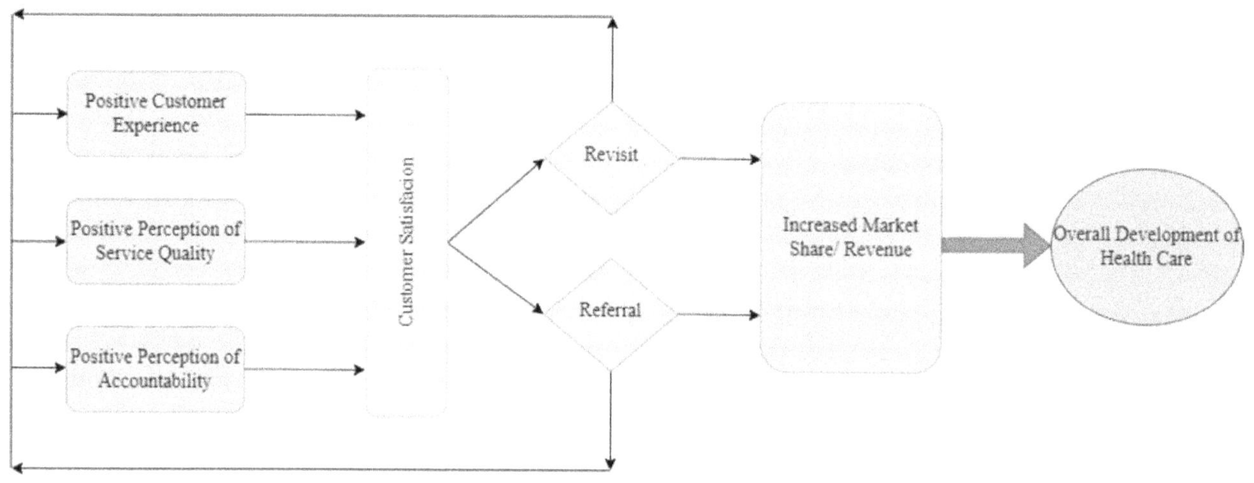

Source: Author's compilation

Figure 5.3: **Road map to increase market share/revenue in diagnostic centre**

This study acknowledges the significance of customer experience and consumer perception, which makes it useful not only for academics but also for practitioners. Organizations can utilize it as a foundation to improve customer experiences and perceptions by using the road map or blueprint (shown in Figure 5.3). As a result, the consumer base will grow and improve. If this is resolved quickly and successfully, a competitive advantage may be obtained. This research emphasizes the importance of shifting attention from traditional service-related concerns to service delivery system designs. Diagnostic centres can generate great patient experiences, increase patient trust, and contribute to better healthcare outcomes by focusing on enhancing the highlighted aspects of customer experience, service quality, and accountability and addressing the contributing factors.

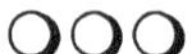

References

Aagja, J. P., & Garg, R. (2010). Measuring perceived service quality for public hospitals (PubHosQual) in the Indian context. International Journal of Pharmaceutical and Healthcare Marketing, 4(1), 60-83.

Abdallah, A. A. (2020). Healthcare engineering: A Lean management approach. Journal of Healthcare Engineering, 2020.

Agarwal, S., Singh, R., Pandiya, B., & Bordoloi, D. (2024). Unveiling the Negative Customer Experience in Diagnostic Centers: A Data Mining Approach. Journal of Multidisciplinary Healthcare, 1491-1504.

Agarwal, S., & Singh, R. (2023). Customers' Perception Towards Accountability of Diagnostic Centres: Evidence from India. Journal of Multidisciplinary Healthcare, 2947-2961.

Agarwal, S., Singh, R., & Upadhyay, C. K. (2022). Service Quality in the Healthcare Industry: A Literature Review and Research Agenda. International Journal of Marketing & Business Communication, 11(1).

Agrawal, R. and Srikant, R., (1994, September). Fast algorithms for mining association rules. In Proc. 20th int. conf. very large data bases, VLDB (Vol. 1215, pp. 487-499).

Agrawal, R., & Srikant, R. Fast algorithms for mining association rules. Proc. 20th int. conf. very large databases, VLDB. 1994; 1215:487-499.

Al-Ababneh, M., Alrowwad, A., & Al-Hussaini, A. (2018). The impact of service quality on patients' satisfaction in the private hospitals in Jordan. International Journal of Marketing Studies, 10(2), 68-84.

Al-Borie, H. M., & Sheikh Damanhouri, A. M. (2013). Patients' satisfaction of service quality in Saudi hospitals: a SERVQUAL analysis. International journal of health care quality assurance, 26(1), 20-30. doi: 10.1108/09526861311288613.

Ali, J., Jusoh, A., Idris, N., & Nor, K. M. (2024). Healthcare service quality and patient satisfaction: a conceptual framework. International Journal of Quality & Reliability Management, 41(2), 608-627.

Ali, J., Jusoh, A., Idris, N., Nor, K. M., Wan, Y., Abbas, A. F., & Alsharif, A. H. (2023). Applicability of healthcare service quality models and dimensions: future research directions. The TQM Journal, 35(6), 1378-1393.

Alizadeh, S., Chavan, M., & Hamin, H. (2016). Quality of care and patient satisfaction amongst Caucasian and non-Caucasian patients: a mixed-method study in Australia. International Journal of Quality & Reliability Management, 33(3), 298-320.

Almsalam, S. (2014). The effects of customer expectation and perceived service quality on customer satisfaction. International Journal of Business and Management Invention, 3(8), 79-84.

Al-Neyadi, H. S., Abdallah, S., & Malik, M. (2018). Measuring patient's satisfaction of healthcare services in the UAE hospitals: Using SERVQUAL. International Journal of Healthcare Management, 11(2), 96-105.

Alolayyan, M. N., & Alfaraj, H. M. (2021). The relationship between emotion and physical environment on the patient'overall satisfaction in the jordanian outpatient private clinics. Academy of Strategic Management Journal, 20(6).

Al-Omar, L. T., Anderson, S. L., Cizmic, A. D., & Vlasimsky, T. B. (2019). Implementation of a pharmacist-led diabetes management protocol. American Health & Drug Benefits, 12(1), 14.

AlOmari, F. (2021). Measuring gaps in healthcare quality using SERVQUAL model: challenges and opportunities in developing countries. Measuring Business Excellence, 25(4), 407-420.

Alrubaiee, L., & Alkaa'ida, F. (2011). The mediating effect of patient satisfaction in the patients' perceptions of healthcare quality-patient trust relationship. International Journal of Marketing Studies, 3(1), 103-123.

Alrubaiee, L., & Alkaa'ida, F. (2021). The relationship between healthcare service quality and patient satisfaction: A systematic review. International Journal of Health Care Quality Assurance, 34(6), 884-898.

Amabile T. (1998). How to kill creativity. Harv Bus Rev 76(5), 76–87

Amjeriya, D., & Kumar Malviya, R. (2012). Measurement of Service Quality. In: Healthcare Organization Student-ujjain engineering college Ujjain. https://www.ijert.org/research/measurement-of-service-quality-in-healthcare-organization-IJERTV1IS8003.pdf

Ampofo, H. (2015). Patient satisfaction with the quality of health care services provided by selected health facilities within cape coast metropolis, Ghana (Doctoral dissertation, University of Cape Coast).

Ancarani, A., Di Mauro, C., & Giammanco, M. D. (2009). The impact of managerial and organizational aspects on hospital wards' efficiency: Evidence from a case study. European Journal of Operational Research, 194(1), 280-293.

Anderson, E. A. (1995). Measuring service quality at a university health clinic. International journal of health care quality assurance, 8(2), 32-37.

Arrow, K. J. (1978). Uncertainty and the welfare economics of medical care. In: Uncertainty in economics (pp. 345-375). Academic Press.

Ayyoubzadeh, S. M., Ghazisaeedi, M., Rostam Niakan Kalhori, S., Hassaniazad, M., Baniasadi, T., Maghooli, K., & Kahnouji, K. (2020). A study of factors related to patients' length of stay using data mining techniques in a general hospital in southern Iran. Health information science and systems, 8, 1-11.

Azam, M., Rahman, Z., Talib, F., & Singh, K. J. (2012). A critical study of quality parameters in health care establishment: developing an integrated quality model. International journal of health care quality assurance, 25(5), 387-402. doi: 10.1108/09526861211235892.

Azman, A., Omar, N. A., & Zainuddin, N. (2022). Service quality and patient satisfaction in healthcare: A systematic literature review. International Journal of Recent Technology and Engineering, 11(2), 374-382.

Babakus, E., & Mangold, W. G. (1992). Adapting the SERVQUAL scale to hospital services: an empirical investigation. Health services research, 26(6), 767.

Babbie, E. R. (2020). The practice of social research. Cengage AU.

Baek, H., Cho, M., Kim, S., Hwang, H., Song, M., & Yoo, S. (2018). Analysis of length of hospital stay using electronic health records: A statistical and data mining approach. PloS one, 13(4), e0195901.

Bagozzi, R. P. (1984). A prospectus for theory construction in marketing. Journal of marketing, 48(1), 11-29.

Bakalikwira, L., Bananuka, J., Kaawaase Kigongo, T., Musimenta, D., & Mukyala, V. (2017). Accountability in the public health care systems: A developing economy perspective. Cogent Business & Management, 4(1), 1334995.

Banasiewicz, A. (2004). Acquiring high value, retainable customers. Journal of Database Marketing & Customer Strategy Management, 12(1), 21-31.

Baranova, P. (2016). Understanding the customer journey through the prism of service design methodology. Routledge.

Batalden, P. B., & Davidoff, F. (2007). What is "quality improvement" and how can it transform healthcare? BMJ Quality & Safety, 16(1), 2-3.

Bavoria, S., Nongkynrih, B., & Krishnan, A. (2019). Health workforce availability and competency to manage noncommunicable diseases at secondary care level hospitals of Delhi. International Journal of Noncommunicable Diseases, 4(2), 38-42.

Bearman, G. M., & Vokes, R. A. (2019). Averting a betrayal of trust: system and individual accountability in healthcare infection prevention. Infection Control & Hospital Epidemiology, 40(8), 918-919.

Becker, L., & Jaakkola, E. (2020). Customer experience: fundamental premises and implications for research. Journal of the Academy of Marketing Science, 48, 630-648.

Berry, L. L. (1988). SERVQUAL: A multiple-item scale for measuring consumer perceptions of service quality. Journal of Retailing, 64(1), 12-40.

Berry, L. L., & Parasuraman, A. (1997). Listening to the customer--the concept of a service-quality information system. MIT Sloan Management Review, 38(3), 65.

Bielawa, A., Frąś, J., & Gołębiowski, M. (2009). Metoda servqual jako skuteczne narzędzie oceny jakości usług. Studia i prace wydziału nauk ekonomicznych i zarządzania, 12, 217-224.

Bitner, M. J., Zeithaml, V. A., & Gremler, D. D. (2020). Services Marketing: Integrating Customer Focus Across the Firm. McGraw-Hill Education.

Black B. The application of SERVQUAL in a district nursing service. Scotland: PTM Publishers; 2000.

Black, J. A., Smith, Y. S., & Keels, J. K. (2014). The Millennial generation and personal accountability: Spiritual and classroom implications. Christian Business Academy Review, 9.

Blagescu, M., de Las Casas, L., & Lloyd, R. (2005). Pathways to accountability. The GAP Framework. Retrieved on November, 19, 2019.

Bland, J. M., & Altman, D. G. (1997). Statistics notes: Cronbach's alpha. Bmj, 314(7080), 572.

Blasco-Arcas, L., Hernandez-Ortega, B., & Jimenez-Martinez, J. (2014). The online purchase as a context for co-creating experiences. Drivers of and consequences for customer behavior. Internet Research, 24(3), 393-412.

Borishade, T., Kehinde, O., Iyiola, O., Olokundun, M., Ibidunni, A., Dirisu, J. and Omotoyinbo, C. (2018). Dataset on customer experience and satisfaction in healthcare sector of Nigeria. Data in brief, 20, 1850-1853.

Boshoff, C., & Gray, B. (2004). The relationships between service quality, customer satisfaction and buying intentions in the private hospital industry. South African journal of business management, 35(4), 27-37.

Bovens, M. (2007). Analysing and assessing accountability: A conceptual framework 1. European law journal, 13(4), 447-468.

Bovens, M. A. P., Goodin, R. E., & Schillemans, T. (Eds.). (2014). The Oxford handbook public accountability. Oxford handbooks.

Boydell, V., Schaaf, M., George, A., Brinkerhoff, D. W., Van Belle, S., & Khosla, R. (2019). Building a transformative agenda for accountability in SRHR: lessons learned from SRHR and accountability literatures. Sexual and reproductive health matters, 27(2), 64-75.

Boysen, P. G. (2013). Just culture: a foundation for balanced accountability and patient safety. Ochsner Journal, 13(3), 400-406.

Brady, M K, Cronin, J and Brand, R R. (2002). "Performance–Only Measurement of Service Quality: A Replication and Extension," Journal of Business Research, 55(1), 17-31.

Brady, M. K., & Cronin Jr, J. J. (2001). Some new thoughts on conceptualizing perceived service quality: a hierarchical approach. Journal of Marketing, 65(3), 34-49.

Brandon-Jones, A., & Silvestro, R. (2010). Measuring internal service quality: comparing the gap-based and perceptions-only approaches. International Journal of Operations & Production Management, 30(12), 1291-1318.

Brandrud, A. S., Schreiner, A., Hjortdahl, P., Helljesen, G. S., Nyen, B., & Nelson, E. C. (2011). Three success factors for continual improvement in healthcare: an analysis of the reports of improvement team members. BMJ Quality & Safety, 20(3), 251-259. doi: 10.1136/bmjqs.2009.038604.

Brandsma, G. J., & Schillemans, T. (2013). The accountability cube: Measuring accountability. Journal of Public Administration Research and Theory, 23(4), 953-975.

Brinkerhoff, D. W. (2003). Accountability and health systems: overview, framework, and strategies. Bethesda, MD: Partners for Health Reformplus Project, Abt Associates.

Brinkerhoff, D. W. (2004). Accountability and health systems: toward conceptual clarity and policy relevance. Health policy and planning, 19(6), 371-379.

Brown, S. W., & Swartz, T. A. (1989). A gap analysis of professional service quality. Journal of marketing, 53(2), 92-98.

Brown, T. J., Churchill Jr, G. A., & Peter, J. P. (1993). Research note: improving the measurement of service quality. Journal of retailing, 69(1), 127.

Bryman, A. (2016). Social research methods. Oxford university press.

Büyüközkan, G., & Çifçi, G. (2012). A combined fuzzy AHP and fuzzy TOPSIS-based strategic analysis of electronic service quality in the healthcare industry. Expert systems with applications, 39(3), 2341-2354.

Byju, K. P. M., & Srinivasulu, Y. (2014). Measuring service quality in private healthcare using SERVPERF scale. J Manag Res, 2(1), 337-349.

Camilleri, D., & O'Callaghan, M. (1998). Comparing public and private hospital care service quality. International journal of health care quality assurance, 11(4), 127-133. doi: 10.1108/09526869810216052.

Campbell, M.C. and Winterich, K.P. (2018). A Framework for the Consumer Psychology of Morality in the Marketplace. Journal of Consumer Psychology, 28(2), 167-179.

Carbone, L. P., & Haeckel, S. H. (1994). Engineering customer experiences. Marketing management, 3(3), 8-19.

Carman, J. M. (1990). Consumer perceptions of service quality: an assessment of T. Journal of retailing, 66(1), 33.

Carpenter, C. R., Mudd, P. A., West, C. P., Wilber, E., & Wilber, S. T. (2020). Diagnosing COVID-19 in the emergency department: a scoping review of clinical examinations, laboratory tests, imaging accuracy, and biases. Academic Emergency Medicine, 27(8), 653-670.

Caru, A., &Cova, B. (2003). Revisiting consumption experience: A more humble but complete view of the concept. Marketing theory, 3(2), 267-286

Cavill, S., & Sohail, M. (2005). Improving public urban services through increased accountability. Journal of Professional Issues in Engineering Education and Practice, 131(4), 263-273.

Chakraborty, R., & Majumdar, A. (2011). Measuring consumer satisfaction in health care sector: the applicability of servqual. Researchers World, 2(4), 149.

Chandra, A., and R/ Kumar. (2012). Factors Influencing Indian Individual Investor Behaviour: Survey Evidence. Decision 39(3), 141 – 167

Chen, C.K., Shie, A.J. and Yu, C.H. (2012). A customer-oriented organisational diagnostic model based on data mining of customer-complaint databases. Expert Systems with Applications, 39(1), 786-792.

Cherizard, C. M. D. (2022). Ethical Leadership Effects on Medical Laboratory Personnel Accountability Behaviors (Doctoral dissertation, Walden University).

Choudhury, M., Singh, R., & Saikia, H. (2016). Measuring customer experience in bancassurance: an empirical study. Market-Tržište, 28(1), 47-62.

Christoglou, K., Vassiliadis, C., & Sigalas, I. (2006). Using SERVQUAL and Kano research techniques in a patient service quality survey. World hospitals and health services: the official journal of the International Hospital Federation, 42(2), 21-26.

Cleary, S. M., Molyneux, S., & Gilson, L. (2013). Resources, attitudes and culture: an understanding of the factors that influence the functioning of accountability mechanisms in primary health care settings. BMC health services research, 13, 1-11.

Cochran, W. G. (1977). Sampling techniques. john wiley & sons.

Concannon, T. W., Griffith, J. L., Kent, D. M., Normand, S. L., Newhouse, J. P., Atkins, J.,... & Selker, H. P. (2009). Elapsed time in emergency medical services for patients with cardiac complaints: are some patients at greater risk for delay? Circulation: Cardiovascular Quality and Outcomes, 2(1), 9-15.

Costello, A. B., & Osborne, J. (2019). Best practices in exploratory factor analysis: Four recommendations for getting the most from your analysis. Practical assessment, research, and evaluation, 10(1), 7.

Coulter, R. A., & Ligas, M. (2004). A typology of customer-service provider relationships: the role of relational factors in classifying customers. Journal of Services Marketing, 18(6), 482-493.

Crago MG. Patient safety, Six Sigma and ISO 9000 quality management: a new emphasis on quality management is essential to improve US healthcare; 2010 [cited June 2019]. Available at: https://www.qualitydigest.com/nov00/html/patient.html.

Creswell, J. W., & Creswell, J. D. (2017). Research design: Qualitative, quantitative, and mixed methods approaches. Sage publications.

Cronin, J and Taylor, S A (1992). Measuring Service Quality: A Reexamination and Extension. Journal of Marketing, 56(3), 55-68.

Cronin, J and Taylor, S A (1994). SERVPERF versus SERVQUAL: Reconciling Performance-based and Perceptions– Minus–Expectations Measurement of Service Quality. Journal of Marketing, 58(January), 125-31.

Cronin, J. J., Brady, M. K., & Hult, G. T. M. (2000). Assessing the effects of quality, value, and customer satisfaction on consumer behavioral intentions in service environments. Journal of Retailing, 76(2), 193-218.

Crosby, P. B. (1979). *Quality is free: The art of making quality certain.* New York: McGraw-Hill Book Co.

Cui, G., Wong, M.L., & Wan, X. (2015). Targeting high value customers while under resource constraint: partial order constrained optimization with genetic algorithm. Journal of Interactive Marketing, 29, 27- 37.

Curry, A., & Sinclair, E. (2002). Assessing the quality of physiotherapy services using SERVQUAL. International Journal of health care quality assurance, 15(5), 197-205.

Dabholkar, P A, Shepherd, D C and Thorpe, D I (2000). A Comprehensive Framework for Service Quality: An Investigation of Critical, Conceptual and Measurement Issues through a Longitudinal Study. Journal of Retailing, 76(2), 139-73.

Dagger, T. S., & Sweeney, J. C. (2007). Service quality attribute weights: how do novice and longer-term customers construct service quality perceptions? Journal of service research, 10(1), 22-42. http://dx.doi.org/10.1177/1094670507303010

Darzi, M.A., Islam, S.B., Khursheed, S.O. and Bhat, S.A. (2023). Service quality in the healthcare sector: a systematic review and meta-analysis. LBS Journal of Management & Research, 21(1), 13-29. https://doi.org/10.1108/LBSJMR-06-2022-0025.

Das, J., Holla, A., Mohpal, A., & Muralidharan, K. (2016). Quality and accountability in health care delivery: audit-study evidence from primary care in India. American Economic Review, 106(12), 3765-3799.

Davidoff, F. (2011). Heterogeneity: we can't live with it, and we can't live without it. BMJ quality & safety, 20(Suppl 1), i11-i12. doi: 10.1136/bmjqs.2010.046094.

Davis, L. L., & Chesterton, P. (2019). Measuring and managing service quality in healthcare: Review and research directions. Journal of Healthcare Management, 64(6), 361-375.

Day, R. M., Demski, R. J., Pronovost, P. J., Sutcliffe, K. M., Kasda, E. M., Maragakis, L. L.,... & Winner, L. (2018). Operating management system for high reliability: leadership, accountability, learning and innovation in healthcare. Journal of Patient Safety and Risk Management, 23(4), 155-166.

De Geyndt, W. (1995). Managing the Quality of Health Care in Developing Countries. Papers 258, World Bank - Technical Papers.

Dean A. (1999). The applicability of SERVQUAL in different healthcare environments. Health Marketing Quarterly. 16(3), 1–21.

Deber, R. B. (2014). Thinking about accountability. Healthcare Policy, 10(SP), 12.

Deka, P.P., & Devi, M.K. (2017). Problems and Prospects of Development in Guwahati, Assam. In: Sustainable Smart Cities in India (pp. 109-122). Springer, Cham.

Deming, W. E. (1986). *Out of the crisis*. Cambridge, MA: Center for Advanced Engineering Study, Massachusetts Institute of Technology.

Demirag, I., Fırtın, C. E., & Tekin Bilbil, E. (2020). Managing expectations with emotional accountability: making City Hospitals accountable during the COVID-19 pandemic in Turkey. Journal of Public Budgeting, Accounting & Financial Management, 32(5), 889-901.

Denis, J. L. (2014). Accountability in healthcare organizations and systems. Healthcare Policy, 10(SP), 8.

Desai, K. T., Nahar, R., & Bansal, R. K. (2012). Study of patient's opinions in a diagnostic centre to measure patient satisfaction. National Journal of Community Medicine, 3(03), 514-517.

Devkota, H.R., Murray, E., Kett, M. and Groce, N. (2017). Healthcare provider's attitude towards disability and experience of women with disabilities in the use of maternal healthcare service in rural Nepal. Reproductive health, 14(1), 1-14.

Dhagarra, D., Goswami, M., & Kumar, G. (2020). Impact of trust and privacy concerns on technology acceptance in healthcare: an Indian perspective. International journal of medical informatics, 141, 104164.

Donabedian, A. (1966). Evaluating the quality of medical care. The Milbank memorial fund quarterly, 44(3), 166-206.

Donabedian, A. (1980). The definition of quality and approaches to its assessment. Ann Arbor, 1.

Donabedian, A. (1987). Commentary on some studies of the quality of care. Health care financing review, 1987(Suppl), 75.

Donabedian, A. (1988). Quality assessment and assurance: unity of purpose, diversity of means. Inquiry, 173-192.

Donabedian, A. (1988). The quality of care: How can it be assessed? JAMA, 260(12), 1743-1748.

Donabedian, A. (2002). An introduction to quality assurance in health care. Oxford University Press.

Dose, J. J., & Klimoski, R. J. (1995). Doing the right thing in the workplace: Responsibility in the face of accountability. Employee Responsibilities and Rights Journal, 8, 35-56.

Drosos, D., Tsotsolas, N., Zagga, A., Chalikias, M.S., &Skordoulis, M. (2015, September). Multicriteria Satisfaction Analysis Application in the Health Care Sector. In: HAICTA (pp. 737-754).

Duggirala, M., Rajendran, C., & Anantharaman, R. N. (2008). Patient-perceived dimensions of total quality service in healthcare. Benchmarking: An international journal.

Edgman-Levitan, S., & Schoenbaum, S. C. (2021). Patient-centered care: achieving higher quality by designing care through the patient's eyes. Israel Journal of Health Policy Research, 10, 1-5.

Edura Wan Rashid, W., & Kamaruzaman Jusoff, H. (2009). Service quality in health care setting. International journal of health care quality assurance, 22(5), 471-482.

Edvardsson, B. (1998). Service quality improvement. Managing service quality: An International Journal, 8(2), 142-149.

Eiriz V, Figueiredo JA. (2005). Quality evaluation in healthcare services based on customer-provider relationships, Int J Health Care Qual Assur. 18(6), 404-12.

Eisenhardt, K. M., & Graebner, M. E. (2007). Theory building from cases: Opportunities and challenges. Academy of management journal, 50(1), 25-32.

Elster J. (1999). Accountability in Athenian politics. Democracy, accountability, and representation. 253-78.

Emanuel, E. J., & Emanuel, L. L. (1996). What is accountability in health care? Annals of internal medicine, 124(2), 229-239.

Endeshaw, B. (2020). Healthcare service quality-measurement models: a review. Journal of Health Research, 35(2), 106-117.

Engelhardt, M., Krämer, T., Marzini, M., Sansour, T., & Zentel, P. (2020). Communication assessment in people with PIMD. Evaluating the use of the INSENSION Questionnaire–Longform (InQL). Psychoeducational Assessment, Intervention and Rehabilitation, 2(1), 1-14.

EROĞLU, S., & ÖZGÜR, G. (2016). Bir üniversite hastanesinde çalışan servis ve yoğun bakım hemşirelerinde zaman yönetimi. Gümüşhane Üniversitesi Sağlık Bilimleri Dergisi, 5(1), 12-22.

Evans, J. R., & Evans, J. R. (2011). Quality management, organization, and strategy. South-Western Cengage Learning.

Farhana, N., Abdul Mohsin, A. M., & KamalulAriffin S. (2021). Examining the Relationship between Customer Experience and Customer Equity in South Asia's Health Sector. Journal of Entrepreneurship, Business, and Economics, 9(1), 275–301

Fatima, I., Humayun, A., Iqbal, U., & Shafiq, M. (2019). Dimensions of service quality in healthcare: a systematic review of literature. International Journal for Quality in Health Care, 31(1), 11-29.

Feigenbaum AV. Total quality control. New York: McGraw-Hill Book Co.; 1983.

Ferguson, R. J., Paulin, M., & Bergeron, J. (2010). Customer sociability and the total service experience: antecedents of positive word-of-mouth intentions. Journal of service management, 21(1), 25-44.

Field, A. (2013). Discovering statistics using IBM SPSS statistics. sage.

Fix, G.M., VanDeusen Lukas, C., Bolton, R.E., Hill, J.N., Mueller, N., LaVela, S.L. and Bokhour, B.G. (2018). Patient-centred care is a way of doing things: How healthcare employees conceptualize patient-centred care. Health Expectations, 21(1), 300-307.

Flin, R. (2010). Rudeness at work. BMJ, 340.

Folkman Curasi, C., & Norman Kennedy, K. (2002). From prisoners to apostles: a typology of repeat buyers and loyal customers in service businesses. Journal of Services Marketing, 16(4), 322-341.

Foroudi, P., Gupta, S., Sivarajah, U. and Broderick, A. (2018). Investigating the effects of smart technology on customer dynamics and customer experience. Computers in Human Behavior, 80, 271-282.

Forster, A. J., & van Walraven, C. (2012). The use of quality indicators to promote accountability in health care: the good, the bad, and the ugly. Open Medicine, 6(2), e75.

Fox, S. (2000). The online health care revolution: How the web helps Americans Take better care of themselves. A Pew Internet and American Life Project Online Report.

Frink DD, Hall AT, Perryman AA, Ranft AL, Hochwarter WA, Ferris GR, Todd Royle M. Meso-level theory of accountability in organizations. In: Research in personnel and human resources management 2008 Jul 25 (pp. 177-245). Emerald Group Publishing Limited. https://doi.org/10.1016/S0742-7301(08)27005-2

Frink, D. D., & Klimoski, R. J. (2004). Advancing accountability theory and practice: Introduction to the human resource management review special edition. Human resource management review, 14(1), 1-17.

Frow, P. and Payne, A. (2007). Towards the 'perfect'customer experience. Journal of Brand Management, 15(2), 89-101.

Gandomi, A. and Haider, M. (2015). Beyond the hype: Big data concepts, methods, and analytics. International journal of information management, 35(2), 137-144.

Gao, Y., Rasouli, S., Timmermans, H. and Wang, Y. (2018). Trip stage satisfaction of public transport users: A reference-based model incorporating trip attributes, perceived service quality, psychological disposition and difference tolerance. Transportation Research Part A: Policy and Practice, 118, 759-775.

Garattini, L., & Padula, A. (2019). Comment on:'The impact of hospital costing methods on cost-effectiveness analysis: a case study'. Pharmacoeconomics, 37(10), 1301-1302.

Garg, R., Rahman, Z., & Kumar, I. (2010). Evaluating a model for analyzing methods used for measuring customer experience. Journal of Database Marketing & Customer Strategy Management, 17(2), 78-90.

Gentile, C., Spiller, N., & Noci, G. (2007). How to sustain the customer experience: An overview of experience components that co-create value with the customer. European management journal, 25(5), 395-410.

Georgiadou, V.A., & Maditinos, D.I. (2017). Measuring the quality of health services provided at a Greek Public Hospital through patient satisfaction. Case Study: The General Hospital of Kavala. International Journal of Business and Economic Sciences Applied Research, 10(2), 60-72.

Ghauri, P., &Gronhaugh, K. (2010). Research methods in Business studied Financial times Prentice Hall. Harlow, England.

Ghazzawi, A. and Alharbi, B. (2019). Analysis of customer complaints data using data mining techniques. Procedia Computer Science, 163, 62-69.

Ghobadian, A., Speller, S., & Jones, M. (1994). Service quality: concepts and models. International journal of quality & reliability management, 11(9), 43-66. https://www.emerald.com/insight/content/doi/10.1108/02656719410074297/full/html

Ghotbabadi, A. R., Feiz, S., & Baharun, R. (2015). Service quality measurements: a review. International Journal of Academic Research in business and social sciences, 5(2), 267-286.

Gishu, T., Weldetsadik, A. Y., & Tekleab, A. M. (2019). Patients' perception of quality of nursing care; a tertiary center experience from Ethiopia. BMC Nursing, 18(1). https://doi.org/10.1186/s12912-019-0361-z

Globenko, A., & Sianova, Z. (2012). Service quality in healthcare: quality improvement initiatives through the prism of patients' and providers' perspectives.

Goldstein, S. M., Johnston, R., Duffy, J., & Rao, J. (2002). The service concept: the missing link in service design research?.Journal of Operations management, 20(2), 121-134.

Gong, T., & Yi, Y. (2018). The effect of service quality on customer satisfaction, loyalty, and happiness in five Asian countries. Psychology & Marketing, 35(6), 427-442.

Gounaris, S. P. (2005). Trust and commitment influences on customer retention: Insights from business-to-business services. Journal of Business Research, 58(2), 126-140.

Gounaris, S. P., Chatzipanagiotou, K. C., & Chatzoglou, P. (2021). Investigating the effect of service quality on customer satisfaction and behavioral intentions in healthcare. Journal of Hospitality Marketing & Management, 30(3), 373-399.

Graham, B., Bond, R., Quinn, M. and Mulvenna, M. (2018). Using data mining to predict hospital admissions from the emergency department. IEEE Access, 6, 10458-10469.

Grefenstette, G. (1999). Tokenization in Syntactic Wordclass Tagging. In: H. van Halteren (Ed.). Syntactic Wordclass Tagging. Kluwer Academic Publishers, 117-133.

Griffey, R.T. and Bohan, J.S. (2006). Healthcare provider complaints to the emergency department: a preliminary report on a new quality improvement instrument. BMJ Quality & Safety, 15(5), 344-346.

Grönroos, C. (1982). An applied service marketing theory. European journal of marketing, 16(7), 30-41.

Grönroos, C. (2001). The perceived service quality concept–a mistake? Managing Service Quality: An International Journal, 11(3), 150-152.

Grossu-Leibovica, D., & Kalkis, H. (2023). Total quality management tools and techniques for improving service quality and client satisfaction in the healthcare environment: A qualitative systematic review. Management Science Letters, 13(2), 118-123.

Gumber, A., & Kulkarni, V. (2000). Health insurance for informal sector: case study of Gujarat. Economic and Political Weekly, 3607-3613.

Guo, L., Ryan, B., Leditschke, I. A., Haines, K. J., Cook, K., Eriksson, L., & Ramanan, M. (2022). Impact of unacceptable behaviour between healthcare workers on clinical performance and patient outcomes: a systematic review. BMJ quality & safety, 31(9), 679-687

Ha, J. F., & Longnecker, N. (2019). Doctor-patient communication: A review. The Ochsner Journal, 19(1), 38-43.

Habbal, Y. (2011). Patient's satisfaction and medical care service quality. International Journal of Business and Public Administration, 8(2), 95-113.

Habli, Z., AlChamaa, W., Saab, R., Kadara, H., & Khraiche, M. L. (2020). Circulating tumor cell detection technologies and clinical utility: Challenges and opportunities. Cancers, 12(7), 1930.

Haeckel, S. H., Carbone, L. P., & Berry, L. L. (2003). How to lead the customer experience. Marketing Management, 12(1), 18-18.

Hallworth, M. J. (2011). The '70% claim': what is the evidence base? Annals of clinical biochemistry, 48(6), 487-488.

Hamer, L. O. (2006). A confirmation perspective on perceived service quality. Journal of services marketing, 20(4), 219-232. http://dx.doi.org/10.1108/08876040610674571

Handayani, P. W., Hidayanto, A. N., Sandhyaduhita, P. I., & Ayuningtyas, D. (2015). Strategic hospital services quality analysis in Indonesia. Expert Systems with Applications, 42(6), 3067-3078.

Haokip, T. (2015). India's look east policy: Prospects and challenges for Northeast India. Studies in Indian Politics, 3(2), 198-211.

Hair, J. F., Black, W. C., Babin, B. J., Anderson, R. E., & Tatham, R. (2006). Multivariate data analysis. Uppersaddle River.

Hair, J. F., Gabriel, M., & Patel, V. (2014). AMOS covariance-based structural equation modeling (CB-SEM): Guidelines on its application as a marketing research tool. Brazilian Journal of Marketing, 13(2).

Heimerl, F., Lohmann, S., Lange, S., & Ertl, T. (2014, January). Word cloud explorer: Text analytics based on word clouds. In: 2014 47th Hawaii international conference on system sciences (pp. 1833-1842). IEEE.

Hendee, W. R. (2008). Safety and accountability in healthcare from past to present. International Journal of Radiation Oncology* Biology* Physics, 71(1), S157-S161.

Herstein, R., & Gamliel, E. (2006). The role of private branding in improving service quality. Managing Service Quality: An International Journal, 16(3), 306-319.

Hilber, A. M., Blake, C., Bohle, L. F., Bandali, S., Agbon, E., & Hulton, L. (2016). Strengthening accountability for improved maternal and newborn health: A mapping of studies in Sub-Saharan Africa. International Journal of Gynecology & Obstetrics, 135(3), 345-357.

Hoe, J. (2007). Quality service in radiology. Biomedical imaging and intervention journal, 3(3).

Holmlund, M., Van Vaerenbergh, Y., Ciuchita, R., Ravald, A., Sarantopoulos, P., Ordenes, F.V., & Zaki, M. (2020). Customer experience management in the age of big data analytics: A strategic framework. Journal of Business Research, 116, 356-365.

Hosseinifard, M., Naghdi, T., Morales-Narváez, E., & Golmohammadi, H. (2021). Toward smart diagnostics in a pandemic scenario: COVID-19. Frontiers in bioengineering and biotechnology, 9, 510.

Hoyer, W. D., Kroschke, M., Schmitt, B., Kraume, K., & Shankar, V. (2020). Transforming the customer experience through new technologies. Journal of interactive marketing, 51(1), 57-71.

https://aspirecircle.org/wp-content/uploads/2022/01/Diagnostic-report-HLTH.pdf

https://dx.doi.org/10.22617/TCS210057-2

https://health.economictimes.indiatimes.com/news/diagnostics/the-rd-landscape-in-indias-diagnostics-sector-improving-innovation-for-better-healthcare/104774857

https://health.economictimes.indiatimes.com/news/diagnostics/amid-regulatory-issues-diagnostic-chains-bet-on-mom-and-pop-labs-to-expand-presence/71752714

https://www.financialexpress.com/healthcare/diagnostic/the-indian-diagnostic-industry-is-touching-new-heights/3028767/

https://www.sentinelassam.com/more-news/editorial/unlocking-assams-export-potential-492475

Hudadoff P (2009) The customer value proposition: differentiation through the eyes of your customer. Applied Product Marketing LLC

Hutcheson, G.D., & Sofroniou, N. (1999). The multivariate social scientist: Introductory statistics using generalized linear models. Sage.

Ishikawa, K. (1998). What is Total Quality Control. Tradução de Iliana Torres, -Controle de Qualidade Total à maneira japonesa, Editora Campus Ltda, 6.

Ismail, A. R. (2011). Experience marketing: An empirical investigation. Journal of Relationship Marketing, 10(3), 167-201.

Israel, M., & Hay, I. (2006). Research ethics for social scientists. Sage.

Itumalla, R., Acharyulu, G. V. R. K., & Shekhar, B. R. (2014). Development of hospitalqual: a service quality scale for measuring in-patient services in hospital. Operations and Supply Chain Management: An International Journal, 7(2), 54-63.

Iyawa, G.E., Herselman, M., & Botha, A. (2016). Digital health innovation ecosystems: From systematic literature review to conceptual framework. Procedia Computer Science, 100, 244-252.

Iyer R, Muncy JA. (2004). Who do you trust? Market. Health Serv. 26-31.

Jabnoun, N., & Chaker, M. (2003). Comparing the quality of private and public hospitals. Managing Service Quality: An International Journal, 13(4), 290-299.

Jain, P., Mittal, E., & Pahuja, J. (2014). Problems faced by the Health Insurance Policy Holders of Different Public and Private Health Insurance Companies for Settlement of their Claims (Case Study of Punjab). BVIMR Management Edge, 7(1), 39-52.

Jain, R., Aagja, J., & Bagdare, S. (2017). Customer experience–a review and research agenda. Journal of service theory and practice, 27(3), 642-662.

Jain, V., Maheshwari, V., & Kaur, P. (2021). An empirical study on healthcare service quality and patient satisfaction: Role of empathy and patient involvement. International Journal of Healthcare Management, 14(1), 24-37.

Jeffrey, L.M., Milne, J., Suddaby, G. and Higgins, A. (2014). Blended learning: How teachers balance the blend of online and classroom components. Journal of Information Technology Education, 13, 121-140

Johnson, C., & Mathews, B. P. (1997). The influence of experience on service expectations. International Journal of Service Industry Management, 8(4), 290-305.

Johnston, R., & Clark, G. (2005). Service operations management: improving service delivery. Pearson Education.

Johnston, R., & Kong, X. (2011). The customer experience: a road-map for improvement. Managing Service Quality: An International Journal, 21(1), 5-24.

Jonkisz, A., Karniej, P., & Krasowska, D. (2021). SERVQUAL Method as an "Old New" Tool for Improving the Quality of Medical Services: A Literature Review. International journal of environmental research and public health, 18(20), 10758. https://doi.org/10.3390/ijerph182010758

Joss, R., & Kogan, M. (1995). Advancing quality: Total quality management in the National Health Service. Open university press.

Jugwanth, B. and Vigar-Ellis, D. (2013). Customer complaint behaviour and companies' recovery initiatives: the case of the hello peter website. Ellis, 20, 143-165.

Jun, M., Peterson, R. T., & Zsidisin, G. A. (1998). The identification and measurement of quality dimensions in health care: focus group interview results. Health care management review, 23(4), 81-96. doi: 10.1097/00004010-199810000-00007.

Juran, J. M., & Gryna, F. M. (1988). Juran's quality control. Handbook. 4ème éd. New York.

Juwaheer, T. D., & Kassean, H. (2006). Exploring quality perceptions of health care operations: a study of public hospitals of Mauritius. Journal of hospital marketing & public relations, 16(1-2), 89-111.

Kaini, B. K. (2013). Healthcare governance for accountability and transparency. Journal of Nepal Health Research Council.

Kaiser, H.F. (1974). An index of factorial simplicity. Psychometrika, 39(1), 31-36.

Kajol, K., Nath, M., Singh, R., Singh, H. R., & Das, A. K. (2020). Factors affecting seasonality in the stock market: A social network analysis approach. International Journal of Accounting & Finance Review, 5(4), 39-59.

Kanis, J., & Müller, L. (2005, September). Automatic lemmatizer construction with focus on OOV words lemmatization. In International Conference on Text, Speech and Dialogue (pp. 132-139). Berlin, Heidelberg: Springer Berlin Heidelberg.

Karimov, Z., & Lee, J. (2020). Determinants of customer satisfaction in the healthcare industry: Evidence from Uzbekistan. International Journal of Quality & Reliability Management, 37(7), 1474-1490.

Kashif, M., Samsi, S.Z.M., Awang, Z. and Mohamad, M. (2016). EXQ: measurement of healthcare experience quality in Malaysian settings: A contextualist perspective. International Journal of Pharmaceutical and Healthcare Marketing, 10(1).

Kassim, N M and Bojei, J (2002). Service Quality: Gaps in the Telemarketing Industry. Journal of Business Research, 55(11), 845-52.

Kaur, M., & Singh, H. (2019). Service quality and patient satisfaction in healthcare: A review. Management in Healthcare, 4(2), 78-88.

Kawaf, F. and Istanbulluoglu, D. (2019). Online fashion shopping paradox: The role of customer reviews and facebook marketing. Journal of Retailing and Consumer Services, 48, 144-153.

Keel, J. (2006). Toolkit, glossary state of Texas State classification. Retrieved from http://www.hr.state.tx.us/workforce/glossary.html

Kerkvoorden, D. V., Ettema, R., & Minkman, M. (2022). Accountability in healthcare in the Netherlands: A scoping review.

Khajehali, N. and Alizadeh, S. (2017). Extract critical factors affecting the length of hospital stay of pneumonia patient by data mining (case study: an Iranian hospital). Artificial intelligence in medicine, 83, 2-13.

Khan, M. N., Rahman, M. M., & Islam, M. R. (2020). Service quality and patient satisfaction in healthcare: A systematic literature review. Management Science Letters, 10(8), 1733-1746.

Khiavi, F. F., Qoliour, M., Saadati, M., Dashtinejad, Z., & Mirr, I. (2018). Gap analysis between expectation-perception of service quality–patients' viewpoint. Journal of Behavioral Health, 7(2), 53-60.

Kıdak, L. B. (2011). Hastane yöneticilerinin zaman yönetimi tutumlarının belirlenmesi: İzmir ili eğitim ve araştırma hastaneleri uygulaması. Selçuk Üniversitesi Sosyal Bilimler Enstitüsü Dergisi, (25), 159-172.

Kilbourne, W. E., Duffy, J. A., Duffy, M., & Giarchi, G. (2004). The applicability of SERVQUAL in cross-national measurements of health-care quality. Journal of services Marketing, 18(7), 524-533.

Kim, T. K. (2015). T test as a parametric statistic. Korean journal of anesthesiology, 68(6), 540.

Kim, H. W., Xu, Y., & Koh, J. (2004). A comparison of online trust building factors between potential customers and repeat customers. Journal of the association for information systems, 5(10), 13.

Kim, H., & So, K. K. F. (2022). Two decades of customer experience research in hospitality and tourism: A bibliometric analysis and thematic content analysis. International Journal of Hospitality Management, 100, 103082.

Kirkland, A. and Hyman, M. (2021). Civil rights as patient experience: How healthcare organizations handle discrimination complaints. Law & Society Review, 55(2), 273-295.

Klaus, P. P., & Maklan, S. (2013). Towards a better measure of customer experience. International journal of market research, 55(2), 227-246.

Kothari, C. R. (2004). Research methodology: Methods and techniques. New Age International.

Kraus, S., Breier, M., & Dasí-Rodríguez, S. (2020). The art of crafting a systematic literature review in entrepreneurship research. International Entrepreneurship and Management Journal, 16(3), 1023–1042. https://doi.org/10.1007/s11365-020-00635-4

Krejcie, R. V., & Morgan, D. W. (1970). Determining sample size for research activities. Educational and psychological measurement, 30(3), 607-610.

Kurnia, Y., Isharianto, Y., Giap, Y. C., & Hermawan, A. (2019, March). Study of application of data mining market basket analysis for knowing sales pattern (association of items) at the O! Fish restaurant using apriori algorithm. In: Journal of Physics: Conference Series (Vol. 1175, No. 1, p. 012047). IOP Publishing.

Kurtuluş, S. A., & Cengiz, E. (2022). Customer experience in healthcare: literature review. Istanbul Business Research, 51(1), 291-312.

Kushwaha, A. K., Kumar, P., & Kar, A. K. (2021). What impacts customer experience for B2B enterprises on using AI-enabled chatbots? Insights from Big data analytics. Industrial Marketing Management, 98, 207-221.

Kwon, H.W., Lee, H. and Ahn, E.K. (2018). National healthcare service and its big data analytics. Healthcare Informatics Research, 24(3), 247-249.

Ladhari, R. (2009). A review of twenty years of SERVQUAL research. International journal of quality and service sciences, 1(2), 172-198.

Lakens, D. (2022). Sample size justification. Collabra: psychology, 8(1), 33267.

Lam, S. K., Sleep, S., Hennig-Thurau, T., Sridhar, S., & Saboo, A.R. (2017). Leveraging frontline employees' small data and firm-level big data in frontline management: An absorptive capacity perspective. Journal of Service Research, 20(1), 12-28

Lee D. (2018). Strategies for technology-driven service encounters for patient experience satisfaction in hospitals. Technol Forecast Soc Chang 137(12), 118–127

Lee, D. (2019). A model for designing healthcare service based on the patient experience. International Journal of Healthcare Management, 12(3), 180-188.

Lee, D., & Kim, K. K. (2017). Assessing healthcare service quality: a comparative study of patient treatment types. International Journal of Quality Innovation, 3(1). https://doi.org/10.1186/s40887-016-0010-5

Lee, D., & Yoon, S. N. (2021). Application of artificial intelligence-based technologies in the healthcare industry: Opportunities and challenges. International Journal of Environmental Research and Public Health, 18(1), 271.

Lee, H., Delene, L. M., Bunda, M. A., & Kim, C. (2000). Methods of measuring health-care service quality. Journal of business research, 48(3), 233-246.

Lee, S. M., & Lee, D. (2022). Effects of healthcare quality management activities and sociotechnical systems on internal customer experience and organizational performance. Service Business, 16(1), 1-28.

Lee, S. M., Lee, D., & Kang, C. Y. (2012). The impact of high-performance work systems in the health-care industry: employee reactions, service quality, customer satisfaction, and customer loyalty. The Service Industries Journal, 32(1), 17-36.

Leedy, P. D., & Ormrod, J. E. (2023). Practical Research: Planning and Design. Pearson.

Lefebvre, B., (2010). Hospital chains in India: the coming of age?

Lekwijit, S., Terwiesch, C., Asch, D. A., & Volpp, K. G. (2023). Evaluating the Efficacy of Connected Healthcare: An Empirical Examination of Patient Engagement Approaches and Their Impact on Readmission. Management Science.

Leninkumar, V. (2017). The relationship between customer satisfaction and customer trust on customer loyalty. International Journal of Academic Research in Business and Social Sciences, 7(4), 450-465.

Lenka, S., Parida, V. and Wincent, J. (2017). Digitalization capabilities as enablers of value co-creation in servitizing firms. Psychology & marketing, 34(1), 92-100.

Levine AS, Plume SK, Nelson EC. (1997) Transforming patient feedback into strategic actions plans. Qual Manag Health Care; 5(3), 28–40

Levy, P. S., & Lemeshow, S. (2013). Sampling of populations: methods and applications. John Wiley & Sons.

Lewis, B (1991). Service Quality: An International Comparison of Bank Customer's Expectations and Perceptions. Journal of Marketing Management, 7(1), 47-62.

Lewis, R C (1987). "The Measurement of Gaps in the Quality of Hotel Service," International Journal of Hospitality Management, 6(2), 83-88.

Li, J., Zhu, X., & Li, J. (2022). The effect of healthcare service quality on patient satisfaction, trust, and loyalty: A meta-analysis. International Journal of Environmental Research and Public Health, 19(1), 220.

Lin, J.W., Thanh, T.D. and Chang, R.G. (2022). Multi-channel word embeddings for sentiment analysis. Soft Computing, 1-13.

Liu, B., Hsu, W., & Ma, Y. (1999). Mining association rules with multiple minimum supports. Proceedings of the fifth ACMSIGKDD international conference on knowledge discovery and data mining. 337–341.

Liu, H., Christiansen, T., Baumgartner, W. A., & Verspoor, K. (2012). BioLemmatizer: a lemmatization tool for morphological processing of biomedical text. Journal of biomedical semantics. 3(1),1-29.

Lohr, S. L. (2021). Sampling: design and analysis. Chapman and Hall/CRC.

Longbottom D, Hilton J. (2011). Service improvement: lessons from the UK financial service sector, International Journal of Quality and Service Sciences. 3(1), 39-59.

Lonial S, Menezes D, Tarim M, Tatoglu E, Zaim S. (2010). An evaluation of SERVQUAL and patient loyalty in an emerging country context, Total Qual. Manag. 21(8), 813-827.

Lopez-Valeiras E, Gomez-Conde J, Lunkes R (2018). Employee reactions to the use of management control systems in hospitals: motivation vs. threat. Gac Sanit. 32(2), 129–134

Lupo, T. (2016). A fuzzy framework to evaluate service quality in the healthcare industry: An empirical case of public hospital service evaluation in Sicily. Applied Soft Computing, 40, 468-478. https://doi.org/10.1016/j.asoc.2015.12.010.

Magatef, S. G. (2015). The impact of tourism marketing mix elements on the satisfaction of inbound tourists to Jordan. International Journal of Business and Social Science, 6(7), 41-58.

Magliocca, N. R., Ellis, E. C., Allington, G. R., De Bremond, A., Dell'Angelo, J., Mertz, O.,... & Verburg, P. H. (2018). Closing global knowledge gaps: Producing generalized knowledge from case studies of social-ecological systems. Global environmental change, 50, 1-14.

Malhotra NK, Ulgado FM, Agarwal J, Baalbaki, IB. (1994). International services marketing: a comparative evaluation of the dimensions of service quality between developed and developing countries, Int. Market. Rev. 11(2), 5-15.

Manary MP, Boulding W, Staelin R, Glickman SW. The patient experience and health outcomes, N Engl J Med. 2013 Jan 17; 368(3): 201-3. doi: 10.1056/NEJMp1211775. Epub 2012 Dec 26.

Mansbridge J. A contingency theory of accountability.

Mascarenhas, O. A., Kesavan, R., & Bernacchi, M. (2006). Lasting customer loyalty: a total customer experience approach. Journal of consumer marketing, 23(7), 397-405.

Maxwell, J. A. (2012). Qualitative research design: An interactive approach. Sage publications.

McColl-Kennedy, J. R., Vargo, S. L., Dagger, T. S., Sweeney, J. C., & Kasteren, Y. V. (2012). Health care customer value cocreation practice styles. Journal of service research, 15(4), 370-389.

McFadden, K. L., Henagan, S. C., & Gowen III, C. R. (2009). The patient safety chain: Transformational leadership's effect on patient safety culture, initiatives, and outcomes. Journal of Operations Management, 27(5), 390-404.

McLaughlin, C. P., & Kaluzny, A. D. (2006). Continuous quality improvement in health care: theory, implementations, and applications. Jones & Bartlett Learning.

Meesala, A. and Paul, J. (2018). Service quality, consumer satisfaction and loyalty in hospitals: Thinking for the future. Journal of Retailing and Consumer Services, 40, 261-269.

Mei, X.Y., Bagaas, I.K. and Relling, E.K. (2019). Customer complaint behaviour (CCB) in the retail sector: why do customers voice their complaints on Facebook? The International Review of Retail, Distribution and Consumer Research, 29(1), 63-78.

Merchant, K. A., & Otley, D. T. (2006). A review of the literature on control and accountability. Handbooks of management accounting research, 2, 785-802.

Meyer, C., & Schwager, A. (2007). Understanding customer experience. Harvard business review, 85(2), 1-11.

Miller, H. D. (2014). Measuring and assigning accountability for healthcare spending. Center for Healthcare Quality and Payment Reform.

Ministry of Health and Family Welfare, Government of India. (2016). National Health Policy 2017. Retrieved from https://www.nhp.gov.in/NHPfiles/national_health_policy_2017.pdf

Miranda, F. J., Chamorro, A., Murillo, L. R., & Vega, J. (2010). Assessing primary healthcare services quality in Spain: managers vs. patients' perceptions. The Service Industries Journal, 30(13), 2137-2149.

Mitropoulos, P., Vasileiou, K. and Mitropoulos, I. (2018). Understanding quality and satisfaction in public hospital services: A nationwide inpatient survey in Greece. Journal of Retailing and Consumer Services, 40, 270-275.

Mohammad Mosadeghrad, A. (2013). Healthcare service quality: towards a broad definition. International journal of health care quality assurance, 26(3), 203-219.

Mohanty, S., & Pattnaik, P. (2020). Measurement and analysis of healthcare service quality: A review. International Journal of Quality & Reliability Management, 37(4), 998-1017.

Mohi, Z. B. (2012). An analysis of restaurant patrons' experiences in Malaysia: a comprehensive hierarchical modelling approach (Doctoral dissertation, Lincoln University).

Moncrieffe, J. (2011). Relational accountability: complexities of structural injustice. Bloomsbury Publishing.

Moraes, C., Cardozo, P. L., & Leal, S. (2021). Service quality in healthcare: A systematic review. International Journal of Health Care Quality Assurance, 34(2), 250-266.

Morse, A. R. (2021). The Importance of Patients' Perspectives in Providing Ophthalmic Care—Lessons From the COVID-19 Pandemic. JAMA Ophthalmology. https://doi.org/10.1001/jamaophthalmol.2021.0121

Mosadeghrad A. M. (2012). A conceptual framework for quality of care. Materia socio-medica, 24(4), 251–261. https://doi.org/10.5455/msm.2012.24.251-261

Mosadeghrad, A. M. (2014a). Factors Affecting Medical Service Quality. Iranian Journal of Public Health, 43(2), 210–220. https://www.ncbi.nlm.nih.gov/pmc/articles/PMC4450689/

Mosadeghrad, A. M. (2014b). Factors influencing healthcare service quality. International journal of health policy and management, 3(2), 77.

Mukinda, F. K., Van Belle, S., & Schneider, H. (2020). Perceptions and experiences of frontline health managers and providers on accountability in a South African health district. International journal for equity in health, 19, 1-11.

Mulgan, R. (2000). 'Accountability': an ever-expanding concept? Public administration, 78(3), 555-573.

Mulyana, D., Soeaidy, M. S., & RahmatTaufiq, A. (2017). Building Customer Trust Through Experience on Healthcare Industry. Advanced Science Letters, 23(9), 9224-9226.

Myers J. (2012). Going above and beyond: improving internal customer satisfaction. Infect Control Today 2012, 1–5

Naidu, A. (2009). Factors affecting patient satisfaction and healthcare quality. International journal of health care quality assurance. 22(4), 366 – 381

Nam, J.H. and Lee, T.J. (2011). Foreign travelers' satisfaction with traditional Korean restaurants. International Journal of Hospitality Management, 30(4), 982-989.

Nambiar, S. (2018). India's Connectivity with ASEAN: What Role for Northeast India? Mainstreaming the Northeast in India's look and act east policy, 131-158.

Nat Natarajan, R. (2006). Transferring best practices to healthcare: opportunities and challenges. The TQM Magazine, 18(6), 572-582.

Naveh, E., & Stern, Z. (2005). How quality improvement programs can affect general hospital performance. International Journal of Health Care Quality Assurance, 18(4), 249-270.

Ndruru, R., & Hasugian, P. M. (2020). Determination of data mining application design patterns booking raw food in restaurant fountain with apriori algorithm. Journal Of Computer Networks, Architecture and High Performance Computing, 2(2), 275-285.

Negassa, G. J., & Japee, G. P. (2023). The Effect of Bonding, Responsiveness and Communication on Customer Retention: The Mediating Role of Customer Satisfaction. Journal of Relationship Marketing, 22(2), 115-131.

Neuman, W. L. (2013). Social Research Methods: Qualitative and Quantitative Approaches (7th ed.). Pearson Education.

Newman, K., Maylor, U., & Chansarkar, B. (2001). The nurse retention, quality of care and patient satisfaction chain. International Journal of health care quality assurance, 14(2), 57-68.

Nguyen, N. X., Tran, K., & Nguyen, T. A. (2021). Impact of service quality on in-patients' satisfaction, perceived value, and customer loyalty: A mixed-methods study from a developing country. Patient preference and adherence, 2523-2538.

Nightingale, A. (2020). Implementing collective leadership in healthcare organisations. Nursing standard, 35(2).

Nikitha, G.N., Chandana, C., Neelashree, N., Nisargapriya, J. and Vishwesh, J. (2020). Bank customer complaints analysis using natural language processing and data mining. International Journal of Progressive Research in Science and Engineering, 1(3), 22-25.

Nunes, R., Brandao, C., & Rego, G. (2011). Public accountability and sunshine healthcare regulation. Health Care Analysis, 19, 352-364.

Nunnally JC. Psychometric Theory: 2d Ed. McGraw-Hill; 1978.

Nurunnabi, M., & Islam, S. K. (2012). Accountability in the Bangladeshi privatized healthcare sector. International Journal of Health Care Quality Assurance, 25(7), 625-644.

Nusairat, T., Al-Amoush, H., & Obeidat, B. (2021). The impact of healthcare service quality on patient satisfaction, loyalty, and word-of-mouth: A systematic review and meta-analysis. International Journal of Environmental Research and Public Health, 18(2), 459.

Oakland, J. (2011). Leadership and policy deployment: the backbone of TQM. Total Quality Management & Business Excellence, 22(5), 517-534.

Oliveira, P., & Von Hippel, E. (2011). Users as service innovators: The case of banking services. Research Policy, 40(6), 806-818.

Oliver, R.L. and Swan, J.E. (1989). Consumer perceptions of interpersonal equity and satisfaction in transactions: a field survey approach. Journal of marketing, 53(2), 21-35.

Oliver, R.L. and Swan, J.E. (1989). Equity and disconfirmation perceptions as influences on merchant and product satisfaction. Journal of consumer research, 16(3), 372-383.

Olsen, J. P. (2014). Accountability and ambiguity. The Oxford handbook of public accountability, 106-123.

Olsson, E.M. (2016). Interpersonal complaints regarding cancer care through a gender lens. International Journal of health care quality assurance, 29(6), 687-702

Olsson, L. E., Friman, M., Pareigis, J., & Edvardsson, B. (2012). Measuring service experience: Applying the satisfaction with travel scale in public transport. Journal of Retailing and Consumer Services, 19(4), 413-418.

Omachonu, V.K., & Einspruch, N.G. (2010). Innovation in healthcare delivery systems: a conceptual framework. The Innovation Journal: The Public Sector Innovation Journal, 15(1), 1-20.

Osterman, P. (2017). Who will care for us?: long-term care and the long-term workforce. Russell Sage Foundation.

Ozyurt, B., & Akcayol, M. A. (2021). A new topic modeling-based approach for aspect extraction in aspect-based sentiment analysis: SS-LDA. Expert Systems with Applications, 168, 114231.

P. Pai, Y., & T. Chary, S. (2013). Dimensions of hospital service quality: A critical review: Perspective of patients from global studies. International journal of health care quality assurance, 26(4), 308-340.

Padma, P., Rajendran, C., & Sai, L. P. (2009). A conceptual framework of service quality in healthcare: perspectives of Indian patients and their attendants. Benchmarking: An International Journal, 16(2), 157-191.

Parasuraman, A., Berry, L. L., & Zeithaml, V. A. (1994). Reassessment of expectations as a comparison standard in measuring service quality: Implications for further research. Journal of Marketing, 58(1), 111-124.

Parasuraman, A., Zeithaml, V. A., & Berry, L. L. (1985). A conceptual model of service quality and its implications for future research. Journal of marketing, 49(4), 41-50.

Park, G. W., Kim, Y., Park, K., & Agarwal, A. (2016). Patient-centric quality assessment framework for healthcare services. Technological Forecasting and Social Change, 113, 468-474.

Patton, M. Q. (2014). Qualitative research & evaluation methods (4th edition). sage.

Paul, J., & Criado, A. R. (2020). The art of writing literature review: What do we know and what do we need to know? International business review, 29(4), 101717.

Pawlson, L. G., Torda, P., Roski, J., & O'Kane, M. E. (2005). The role of accreditation in an era of market-driven accountability. Am J Manag Care, 11(5), 290-293.

Payne, A. and Frow, P. (2017). Relationship marketing: looking backwards towards the future. Journal of services marketing, 31(1), 11-15

Petersen, M.B.H. (1988). Measuring patient satisfaction: collecting useful data. Journal of Nursing Care Quality, 2(3), 25-35.

Pighi, L., Henry, B. M., De Nitto, S., Gianfilippi, G., Raschella, N., Salvagno, G. L., & Lippi, G. (2023). Impact of the COVID-19 pandemic on the volume of laboratory testing. biochimica clinica, 47(2), 171.

Pijls, R., Groen, B. H., Galetzka, M., & Pruyn, A. T. (2017). Measuring the experience of hospitality: Scale development and validation. International journal of hospitality management, 67, 125-133.

Pine, K., & Mazmanian, M. (2015). Emerging insights on building infrastructure for data-driven transparency and accountability of organizations. iConference 2015 Proceedings.

Platt, A.W., 2010. Handling complaints. BMJ, 340.

Plisson, J., Lavrac, N. and Mladenic, D. (2004, October). A rule-based approach to word lemmatization. In Proceedings of IS, 3, 83-86.

Ponsignon, F., Smart, A. and Phillips, L. (2018). A customer journey perspective on service delivery system design: insights from healthcare. International Journal of Quality & Reliability Management, 35(10), 2328-2347

Poulsson, S. H., & Kale, S. H. (2004). The experience economy and commercial experiences. The marketing review, 4(3), 267-277.

Powell, D., & Hannah, A. (2024). The dichotomy of diagnostics: exploring the value for consumers, clinicians and care pathways. NPJ Digital Medicine, 7(1), 101.

Prakash, A., & Mohanty, R. P. (2013). Understanding service quality. Production Planning & Control, 24(12), 1050-1065.

Priyadarshi, M., & Kumar, S. (2020). Accountability in healthcare in India. Indian Journal of Community Medicine, 45(2), 125-129.

Psomas, E. L., & Jaca, C. (2016). The impact of total quality management on service company performance: evidence from Spain. International Journal of Quality & Reliability Management, 33(3), 380-398.

Purcărea, V. L., Gheorghe, I. R., & Petrescu, C. M. (2013). The assessment of perceived service quality of public health care services in Romania using the SERVQUAL scale. Procedia Economics and Finance, 6, 573-585.

Putturaj, M., Van Belle, S., Engel, N., Criel, B., Krumeich, A., Nagendrappa, P. B., & Srinivas, P. N. (2021). Multilevel governance framework on grievance redressal for patient rights violations in India. Health policy and planning, 36(9), 1470-1482.

Rao, D., Dhakshaini, M. R., Kurthukoti, A., & Doddawad, V. G. (2018). Biomedical waste management: A study on assessment of knowledge, attitude and practices among health care professionals in a tertiary care teaching hospital. Biomedical and Pharmacology Journal, 11(3), 1737-1743.

Ritchie, J. B., & Hudson, S. (2009). Understanding and meeting the challenges of consumer/tourist experience research. International Journal of Tourism Research, 11(2), 111-126.

Romzek, B. S., & Dubnick, M. J. (2018). Accountability. In Defining public administration, 382-395. Routledge.

Rooney, A. L., & Van Ostenberg, P. R. (1999). Licensure, accreditation, and certification: approaches to health services quality. Bethesda: Center for Human Services, Quality Assurance Project.

Roshnee Ramsaran-Fowdar, R. (2008). The relative importance of service dimensions in a healthcare setting. International journal of health care quality assurance, 21(1), 104-124.

Roy, S., Singh, H. R., & Singh, R. (2017). Factors affecting the financial inclusion of SHG members: An empirical study in Tripura. IUP Journal of Bank Management, 16(3), 59-83

Rudd, R. E., Anderson, J. E., Oppenheimer, S., & Nath, C. (2023). Health literacy: an update of medical and public health literature. In Review of Adult Learning and Literacy, Volume 7 (pp. 175-204). Routledge.

Sadiq Sohail, M. (2003). Service quality in hospitals: more favourable than you might think. Managing Service Quality: An International Journal, 13(3), 197-206.

Sadeghi, T., & Bemani, A. (2011). Assessing the quality of bank services by using the gap analysis model. Asian Journal of Business Management Studies, 2(1), 14-23.

Safdar, S., Khan, S. A., & Shaukat, A. (2019, October). Customer experience management (CEM) for automation, data collection and methodology. In: 2019 International Conference on Information and Communication Technology Convergence (ICTC) (pp. 1354-1358). IEEE.

Samsa, Ç., & Yüce, A. (2022). Understanding customers hospital experience and value co-creation behavior. The TQM Journal, 34(6), 1860-1876.

Sánchez-Bayón, A., González-Arnedo, E., & Andreu-Escario, Á. (2022). Spanish healthcare sector management in the COVID-19 crisis under the perspective of Austrian economics and new-institutional economics. Frontiers in Public Health, 10, 801525.

Satish, L. and Yusof, N. (2017). A review: big data analytics for enhanced customer experiences with crowd sourcing. Procedia computer science, 116, 274-283.

Saunders, M., Lewis, P., & Thornhill, A. (2009). Research methods for business students. Pearson education.

Schedler, A., Diamond, L. J., & Plattner, M. F. (Eds.). (1999). The self-restraining state: power and accountability in new democracies. Lynne Rienner Publishers.

Schiavone, F., Leone, D., Sorrentino, A. and Scaletti, A. (2020). Re-designing the service experience in the value co-creation process: an exploratory study of a healthcare network. Business Process Management Journal. 26(4), 889-908.

Schiavone, F., Leone, D., Sorrentino, A., & Scaletti, A. (2020). Re-designing the service experience in the value co-creation process: an exploratory study of a healthcare network. Business Process Management Journal, 26 (4), 889-908

Schillemans, T. (2013). The public accountability review. A meta-analysis of public accountability research in six academic disciplines.

Senić, V., & Marinković, V. (2013). Patient care, satisfaction and service quality in health care. International journal of consumer studies, 37(3), 312-319.

Seth, N., Deshmukh, S. G., & Vrat, P. (2005). Service quality models: a review. International journal of quality & reliability management, 22(9), 913-949.

Shafiq, M., Naeem, M. A., Munawar, Z., & Fatima, I. (2017). Service Quality Assessment of Hospitals in Asian Context: An Empirical Evidence from Pakistan. INQUIRY: The Journal of Health Care Organization, Provision, and Financing, 54, 004695801771466. https://doi.org/10.1177/0046958017714664

Shehada, A. K., Albelbeisi, A. H., Albelbeisi, A., El Bilbeisi, A. H., & El Afifi, A. (2021). The fear of COVID-19 outbreak among health care professionals in Gaza Strip, Palestine. SAGE open medicine, 9, 20503121211022987.

Sheth, J. N., Jain, V., & Ambika, A. (2023). The growing importance of customer-centric support services for improving customer experience. Journal of Business Research, 164, 113943.

Sieber, J. E. (1998). Planning ethically responsible research. Handbook of applied social research methods, 127-156.

Singh, D., & Dixit, K. (2020). Measuring perceived service quality in healthcare setting in developing countries: A review for enhancing managerial decision-making. Journal of Health Management, 22(3), 472-489.

Singh, R. (2012). Risk perception of Investors in initial public offer of shares: A psychometric study. Asia Pacific Journal of Risk and Insurance, 6(2), 44-56

Singh, R., & Bhattacharjee, J. (2019). Measuring equity share related risk perception of investors in economically backward regions. Risks, 7(1), 12.

Singh, R., &Choudhury, M. (2017). Measuring customers' perception in bancassurance channel using psychometric scale. DLSU Business & Economics Review, 26(2), 1-6.

Singh, R., Agarwal, S. and Pandiya, B. (2022). Customer Experience in Diagnostic Centres: An Empirical Study. Academy of Marketing Studies Journal, 26(3), 1-15.

Singh, R., Agarwal, S. and Singh, N. (2021). Adaptation of Roster Format in Food Joints. Journal of Case Research, 12(1).

Singh, R., Bhattacharjee, J., & Kajol, K. (2024). Factors affecting risk perception in respect of equity shares: a social network analysis approach. Vision, 28(3), 386-399.

Singh, R., Deb, S., Pandiya, B., &Gope, A. (2021). Measuring attitude towards mutual fund investment decisions: evidences from Tripura, India. Indian Journal of Finance and Banking, 8(1), 1-12.

Singh, R., Pandiya, B., Upadhyay, C. K., & Singh, M. K. (2020a). IT-governance framework considering service quality and information security in banks in India. International Journal of Human Capital and Information Technology Professionals (IJHCITP), 11(1), 64-91.

Sittig, D. F., & Singh, H. (2015). A new socio-technical model for studying health information technology in complex adaptive healthcare systems. Cognitive Informatics for Biomedicine: Human Computer Interaction in Healthcare, 59-80.

Skaria, R., Satam, P., & Khalpey, Z. (2020). Opportunities and challenges of disruptive innovation in medicine using artificial intelligence.The American Journal of Medicine, 133(6), e215-e217.

Smith, J., Anderson, S., & Fox, G. (2017). A quality system's impact on the service experience. International Journal of Operations & Production Management, 37(12), 1817-1839.

Smith, R A and Houston, M J (1982). Script-based Evaluations of Satisfaction with Services, in Berry, L, Shostack, G and Upah, G (eds.), Emerging Perspectives on Services Marketing, Chicago: American Marketing Association, 59-62

Snoj, B., & Mumel, D. (2002). The measurement of perceived differences in service quality—The case of health spas in Slovenia. Journal of vacation marketing, 8(4), 362-379.

Snyder, H. (2019). Literature review as a research methodology: An overview and guidelines. Journal of business research, 104, 333-339.

Sohail, M. (2005). Accessibility and quality of government primary health care: achievement and constraints. The Bangladesh Development Studies, 63-98.

Srikant, R., &Agrawal, R. (1995). Mining generalized association rules. IBM Research Division Zurich, 407-419.

Stangl, B., Kastner, M., & Prayag, G. (2017). Pay-what-you-want for high-value priced services: Differences between potential, new, and repeat customers. Journal of business research, 74, 168-174.

Stevens, J. (2002). Applied multivariate statistics for the social sciences (Vol. 4). Mahwah, NJ: Lawrence Erlbaum Associates.

Sumaedi, S., Yarmen, M., & Bakti, I. G. M. Y. (2016). Healthcare service quality model: a multi-level approach with empirical evidence from a developing country. International Journal of Productivity and Performance Management, 65(8), 1007-1024.

Sun, L.N. (2020). An improved apriori algorithm based on support weight matrix for data mining in transaction database. Journal of Ambient Intelligence and Humanized Computing, 11(2), 495-501.

Sureshchandar, G. S., Rajendran, C., & Anantharaman, R. N. (2002). The relationship between management's perception of total quality service and customer perceptions of service quality. Total quality management, 13(1), 69-88.

Sureshchandar, G. S., Rajendran, C., & Kamalanabhan, T. J. (2001). Customer perceptions of service quality: A critique. Total quality management, 12(1), 111-124.

Suri, H. (2011). Purposeful sampling in qualitative research synthesis. Qualitative research journal, 11 (2), 63-75.

Swain, S., & Kar, N. C. (2018). Hospital service quality as antecedent of patient satisfaction–a conceptual framework. International Journal of Pharmaceutical and Healthcare Marketing, 12(3), 251-269.

Swanson, K. M. (2015). Kristen Swanson's theory of caring. nursing theories and nursing practice, 521.

Szymanski, D. M., & Henard, D. H. (2001). Customer satisfaction: A meta-analysis of the empirical evidence. Journal of the academy of marketing science, 29(1), 16-35.

Taher, M. (1994). Librarianship and Library Science in India: An Outline of Historical Perspectives (Vol. 60). Concept Publishing Company. New Delhi

Taherdoost, H. (2016). Sampling methods in research methodology; how to choose a sampling technique for research. How to choose a sampling technique for research (April 10, 2016).

Tajpour, M., Hosseini, E., & Salamzadeh, A. (2020). The effect of innovation components on organisational performance: case of the governorate of Golestan Province. International Journal of Public Sector Performance Management, 6(6), 817-830.

Talib, F., Azam, M., & Rahman, Z. (2015). Service quality in healthcare establishments: a literature review. International Journal of Behavioural and Healthcare Research, 5(1-2), 1-24. https://www.inderscienceonline.com/doi/abs/10.1504/IJBHR.2015.071465

Tarmizi, R., Suhada, H., Apriani, D., Hasanudin, M., Kristiadi, D.P., & Hidayat, W. (2021). Customer Experience Management (CEM) Supports the Quality of Hospital Services Based on RFID. In 1st Paris Van Java International Seminar on Health, Economics, Social Science and Humanities (PVJ-ISHESSH 2020) (pp. 688-693). Atlantis Press.

Tavakol, M., & Dennick, R. (2011). Making sense of Cronbach's alpha. International journal of medical education, 2, 53.

Taylor, S. A., & Baker, T. L. (1994). An assessment of the relationship between service quality and customer satisfaction in the formation of consumers' purchase intentions. Journal of Retailing, 70(2), 163-178.

Taymaz, S., Iyigun, C., Bayindir, Z. P., & Dellaert, N. P. (2020). A healthcare facility location problem for a multi-disease, multi-service environment under risk aversion. Socio-Economic Planning Sciences, 71, 100755.

Teas, R. K. (1994). Expectations as a comparison standard in measuring service quality: an assessment of a reassessment. Journal of marketing, 58(1), 132-139.

Tetlock, P. E. (1983). Accountability and complexity of thought. Journal of personality and social psychology, 45(1), 74.

Thomas, P. G. (1998). The changing nature of accountability. Taking stock: Assessing public sector reforms, 2, 348-93.

Thompson, A. G. (1983). The measurement of patients' perceptions of the quality of hospital care. The University of Manchester (United Kingdom).

Trochim, W. M., Donnelly, J. P., & Arora, K. (2016). Research methods: The essential knowledge base. Cengage learning.

Tucker, J.L. (2002). The moderators of patient satisfaction. Journal of Management in Medicine, 16 (1), 48-66

Turner, P.D., & Pol, L.G. (1995). Beyond patient satisfaction. Marketing Health Services, 15(3), 45.

Um, K.H. and Lau, A.K. (2018). Healthcare service failure: how dissatisfied patients respond to poor service quality. International Journal of Operations & Production Management, 38(5), 1245-1270

Upadhyai, R., Upadhyai, N., Jain, A. K., Roy, H., & Pant, V. (2020). Health care service quality: a journey so far. Benchmarking: An International Journal, 27(6), 1893-1927.

van Iwaarden, J., van der Wiele, T., Ball, L., & Millen, R. (2003). Applying SERVQUAL to Web sites: An exploratory study. International Journal of Quality and Reliability Management, 20(8), 919–935.

Vance, A., Lowry, P. B., & Eggett, D. (2013). Using accountability to reduce access policy violations in information systems. Journal of management information systems, 29(4), 263-290.

Vance, A., Lowry, P. B., & Eggett, D. (2015). Increasing accountability through user-interface design artifacts. MIS quarterly, 39(2), 345-366.

Vargo, S. L., & Lusch, R. F. (2008). Service-dominant logic: continuing the evolution. Journal of the Academy of marketing Science, 36, 1-10.

Vaske, J. J., Beaman, J., & Sponarski, C. C. (2017). Rethinking internal consistency in Cronbach's alpha. Leisure sciences, 39(2), 163-173.

Velazquez, B.M., Blasco, M.F., Saura, I.G. and Contri, G.B. (2010). Causes for complaining behaviour intentions: the moderator effect of previous customer experience of the restaurant. Journal of Services Marketing, 24(7), 532–545

Venn, S., & Fone, D. L. (2005). Assessing the influence of socio-demographic factors and health status on expression of satisfaction with GP services. Clinical Governance: An International Journal, 10(2), 118-125.

Veres III, J. G., Locklear, T. S., & Sims, R. R. (1990). Job analysis in practice: a brief review of the role of job analysis in human resources management. Human resource management: Perspectives and issues, 8(5), 79-103.

Verhoef, P. C., Reinartz, W. J., & Krafft, M. (2010). Customer engagement as a new perspective in customer management. Journal of service research, 13(3), 247-252.

Verhoef, P.C., Kannan, P.K. and Inman, J.J. (2015). From multi-channel retailing to omni-channel retailing: introduction to the special issue on multi-channel retailing. Journal of retailing, 91(2), 174-181.

Vianna, L.S. and Wazlawick, R.S. (2020, March). Data Mining for Hospital Morbidity Forecasting. In 2020 IEEE International Conference on Software Architecture Companion (ICSA-C) (pp. 167-172). IEEE.

Vogus, T.J. and McClelland, L.E., 2016. When the customer is the patient: Lessons from healthcare research on patient satisfaction and service quality ratings. Human Resource Management Review, 26(1), 37-49.

Voss, C., Roth, A.V., & Chase, R.B. (2008). Experience, service operations strategy, and services as destinations: foundations and exploratory investigation. Production and operations management, 17(3), 247-266.

Vriens, M., Brokaw, S., Rademaker, D. and Verhulst, R. (2019). The marketing research curriculum: Closing the practitioner–academic gaps. International Journal of Market Research, 61(5), 492-501.

Wachter, R. M. (2013). Personal accountability in healthcare: searching for the right balance. BMJ quality & safety, 22(2), 176-180.

Wang, C. and Zheng, X. (2020). Application of improved time series Apriori algorithm by frequent itemsets in association rule data mining based on temporal constraint. Evolutionary Intelligence, 13(1), 39-49.

Wanjau, K. N., Muiruri, B. W., & Ayodo, E. (2012). Factors affecting the provision of service quality in the public health sector: A case of Kenyatta national hospital.

Wanninayake, W. M. C. B., Jayawardena, C., & Madurapperuma, D. (2017). Factors affecting service quality of public and private hospitals in Colombo district, Sri Lanka. Journal of Health Management, 19(3), 367-383.

Wasike, M. (2020). Determinants of uptake of Health care insurance among households in Kibera Informal settlement, Nairobi County (Doctoral dissertation, JKUAT-COHES).

Weiss, J.N. (2023). What are the Customer Experience Challenges in Healthcare? In: Physician Crisis. Springer, Cham. https://doi.org/10.1007/978-3-031-27979-9_10

Wilbur, W.J. and Sirotkin, K. (1992). The automatic identification of stop words. Journal of information science, 18(1), 45-55.

Wisniewski, M. (1996). Measuring service quality in the public sector: the potential for SERVQUAL. Total quality management, 7(4), 357-366.

Witkowski, T H and Wolfinbarger, M F (2002). Comparative Service Quality: German and American Ratings across Service Settings. Journal of Business Research, 55 (11), 875-81.

Witvliet, C. V., Jang, S. J., Johnson, B. R., Evans, C. S., Berry, J. W., Torrance, A.,... & Bradshaw, M. (2024). Transcendent accountability: Construct and measurement of a virtue that connects religion, spirituality, and positive psychology. The Journal of Positive Psychology, 19(2), 243-256.

Wolf PhD, C. P. X. P., & Jason, A. (2018). Elevating the discourse on experience in healthcare's uncertain times. Patient Experience Journal, 5(3), 1-5.

Worlu, R., Kehinde, O.J. and Borishade, T.T. (2016). Effective customer experience management in health-care sector of Nigeria: a conceptual model. International journal of pharmaceutical and healthcare marketing, 10(4), 449-466.

Wu, T. (2020). From Time Sheets to Tablets: Documentation Technology in Frontline Service Sector Managers' Coordination of Home Healthcare Services. Work and Occupations, 47(3), 378-405.

Xie, G., Qiu, P., Chen, Y., & Song, J. (2007). Expectation and Satisfaction of Rural Tourism: ACase Study of Hainan, China. Ecological Economy, 3, 405-416.

Xu, J., Zhao, J., Zhao, N., Xue, C., Fan, L., Qi, Z. and Wei, Q. (2018, August). The Research and Construction of Complaint Orders Classification Corpus in Mobile Customer Service. In: CCF International Conference on Natural Language Processing and Chinese Computing (pp. 351-361). Springer, Cham.

Yahui Hsieh, S. (2012). Using complaints to enhance quality improvement: developing an analytical tool. International journal of health care quality assurance, 25(5), 453-461.

Yang, Y., Xu, D.L., Yang, J.B. and Chen, Y.W. (2018). An evidential reasoning-based decision support system for handling customer complaints in mobile telecommunications. Knowledge-Based Systems, 162, 202-210.

Yong, A. G., & Pearce, S. (2013). A beginner's guide to factor analysis: Focusing on exploratory factor analysis. Tutorials in quantitative methods for psychology, 9(2), 79-94.

Yoon, S. N., & Lee, D. (2018). Artificial intelligence and robots in healthcare: What are the success factors for technology-based service encounters? International Journal of Healthcare Management.

Yoon, Y. S., & Suh, E. H. (2003). Organizational culture, innovation, and performance: A test of competing models in South Korea. Asia Pacific Journal of Management, 20(4), 503-520.

Young, C, Cunningham, L and Lee, M (1994). Assessing Service Quality as an Effective Management Tool: The Case of the Airline Industry. Journal of Marketing Theory and Practice, 2(Spring), 76-96.

Zabada, C., Rivers, P. A., & Munchus, G. (1998). Obstacles to the application of total quality management in health-care organizations. Total quality management, 9(1), 57-66.

Zainuddin, N., Russell-Bennett, R., & Previte, J. (2013). The value of health and wellbeing: an empirical model of value creation in social marketing. European Journal of Marketing, 47 (9), 1504-1524.

Zeithaml, V. A., Berry, L. L., & Parasuraman, A. (1988). Communication and control processes in the delivery of service quality. Journal of marketing, 52(2), 35-48.

Zeithaml, V. A., Parasuraman, A., & Berry, L. L. (1990). Delivering quality service: Balancing customer perceptions and expectations. Simon and Schuster. New York: The Free Press.

Zhang, M., & He, C. (2010). Survey on association rules mining algorithms. Advancing computing, communication, control and management, 111-118.

Zhang, R., Jun, M., & Palacios, S. (2023). M-shopping service quality dimensions and their effects on customer trust and loyalty: An empirical study. International Journal of Quality & Reliability Management, 40(1), 169-191.

Zineldin, M. (2006). The quality of health care and patient satisfaction: an exploratory investigation of the 5Qs model at some Egyptian and Jordanian medical clinics. International journal of health care quality assurance, 19(1), 60-92.

Zolkiewski, J., Story, V., Burton, J., Chan, P., Gomes, A., Hunter-Jones, P.,... & Robinson, W. (2017). Strategic B2B customer experience management: the importance of outcomes-based measures. Journal of Services Marketing, 31(2), 172-184.

Zou, K., Li, H. Y., Zhou, D., & Liao, Z. J. (2020). The effects of diagnosis-related groups payment on hospital healthcare in China: a systematic review. BMC health services research, 20(1), 1-11.

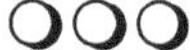

Annexure

Appendix 1

Interview Schedule

PART 'A'

Personal information of the respondent

In this part of the questionnaire, the respondents need to fill the gaps specified in each column. Some columns are optional to fill. If the respondents do not want to disclose the information, they can leave the columns blank.

1. Age: Please (√) the appropriate option

Less than 25 years	
25 years to 35 years	
35 years to 45 years	
45 years to 55 years	
More than 55 years	

2. Gender: Please (√) the appropriate option

Male	
Female	
Others	

3. Marital Status: Please (√) the appropriate option

Married	
Unmarried	
Divorced	
Widow/Widower	
Others	

4. Number of Members in Family: Please (√) the appropriate option

1	2	3	4	5	6	7	8	More than 8

5. Family Income(yearly): Please (√) the appropriate option

Less than 2.5 lakhs	
2.5 lakhs – 5 lakhs	
5 lakhs - 7.5 lakhs	
7.5lakhs – 10 lakhs	
More than 10 lakhs	

6. Education: Please (√) the appropriate option

Less than class 10	
Less than class 12	
Undergraduate	
Graduate	
Post Graduate	
PhD	
Others	

7. Occupation: Please (√) the appropriate option

Professional	
Business	
Service	
Others	

8. Name of the Diagnostic centre/clinic about which you wish to share your experience/opinion

PART 'B'
Customer Experience Questionnaire

Please give your response on a five-point scale concerning the experience you have with the diagnostic centre/clinic that you visited last time. [5] indicate very good experience, [4] indicates good experience, [3] indicates moderate experience, [2] is a bad experience and [1] is a very bad experience. Please tick (√) the appropriate option.

Sl. No.	Particulars					
1	Explaining the process of doing diagnosis	5	4	3	2	1
2	Clarification of doubts raised related to the diagnosis	5	4	3	2	1
3	To suggest the most affordable way of diagnosis	5	4	3	2	1
4	To suggest the most suitable type of diagnosis	5	4	3	2	1
5	Availability of the personnel at the diagnostic centre	5	4	3	2	1
6	Not disclosing your personal information to others	5	4	3	2	1
7	Convenience of paying the requisite fees	5	4	3	2	1
8	Time required to get the report	5	4	3	2	1
9	To provide necessary help after diagnosis is done	5	4	3	2	1
10	Comfort with the way some personal information are asked	5	4	3	2	1
11	Comfort with the type of document sought	5	4	3	2	1
12	Getting help while filling up some forms	5	4	3	2	1
13	Giving Intimation about the time of next check up	5	4	3	2	1
14	Giving information about the time of delivery of report	5	4	3	2	1
15	Online delivery of report	5	4	3	2	1
16	Help in getting insurance settlement	5	4	3	2	1
17	Timely delivery of report	5	4	3	2	1
18	To keep you informed about any regulatory aspect	5	4	3	2	1
19	Eager to solve problems at an earliest.	5	4	3	2	1
20	To give occasional gifts like diaries, calendars etc.	5	4	3	2	1
21	To keep accurate records of previous reports	5	4	3	2	1
22	To tell exactly when the services will be performed	5	4	3	2	1
23	Willingness to provide service do not vary with each counter	5	4	3	2	1
24	giving individual attention	5	4	3	2	1
25	Parking facility	5	4	3	2	1
26	Waiting area	5	4	3	2	1
27	Sitting facility	5	4	3	2	1
28	Ambience	5	4	3	2	1

PART 'C'
Service Quality
EXPECTATION

This survey deals with your opinions of **diagnostic** services. Please show the extent to which you think clinics offering **diagnostic** services should possess the features described by each statement. Do this by picking one of the five numbers next to each statement. If you strongly agree that this clinic should possess a feature, circle 5. If you strongly disagree that this clinic should possess a feature, circle 1. If your feelings are not strong, circle one of the numbers in the middle. There are no right or wrong answers. All we are interested in is the number that best shows your **expectations** about clinics offering **diagnostic** services.

Q1-Q4: Tangibility, Q5-Q9: Reliability, Q10-13: Responsiveness, Q14-17: Assurance, Q18-22: Empathy

S. No.	Items	SA	A	N	D	SD
1	They should have up-to-date equipment	5	4	3	2	1
2	Their physical facilities should be visually appealing	5	4	3	2	1
3	Their employees should be well dressed and appear neat	5	4	3	2	1
4	The appearance of the physical facilities of these clinics should be following the type of services provided	5	4	3	2	1
5	When these clinics promise to do something by a certain time, they should do so	5	4	3	2	1
6	When customers have problems, these clinics should be sympathetic and reassuring	5	4	3	2	1
7	These clinics should be dependable	5	4	3	2	1
8	They should provide their services at the time they promise to do so	5	4	3	2	1
9	They should keep their records accurately	5	4	3	2	1
10	They shouldn't be expected to tell customers exactly when services will be performed	5	4	3	2	1
11	It is not realistic for customers to expect prompt service from the employees of these clinics	5	4	3	2	1
12	Their employees don't always have to be willing to help customers	5	4	3	2	1
13	It is okay if they are too busy to respond to customer requests promptly	5	4	3	2	1
14	Customers should be able to trust the employees of these clinics	5	4	3	2	1
15	Customers should be able to feel safe in their transactions with these firms' employees	5	4	3	2	1
16	Their employees should be polite	5	4	3	2	1
17	Their employees should get adequate support from these clinics to do their jobs well	5	4	3	2	1

S. No.	Items	SA	A	N	D	SD
18	These clinics should not be expected to give customers individual attention	5	4	3	2	1
19	Employees of these clinics cannot be expected to give customers personal attention	5	4	3	2	1
20	It is unrealistic to expect employees to know what the needs of their customers are	5	4	3	2	1
21	It is unrealistic to expect these clinics to have their customer's best interests at heart	5	4	3	2	1
22	They shouldn't be expected to have operating hours convenient to all their customers	5	4	3	2	1

PERCEPTION

This survey deals with your **feelings** about the diagnostic clinic services. Please show the extent to which you think diagnostic clinic services possess the features described by each statement. Do this by picking one of the five numbers next to each statement. If you strongly agree that the clinic possesses a feature, circle 5 and if you strongly disagree that the clinic possesses a feature, circle 1. If your feelings are not strong, circle one of the numbers in the middle. There are no right or wrong answers. All we are interested in is the number that best shows your feelings about your diagnostic clinic.

Q1-Q4: Tangibility, Q5-Q9: Reliability, Q10-13: Responsiveness, Q14-17: Assurance, Q18-22: Empathy

S. No.	Items	SA	A	N	D	SD
1	This clinic has up-to-date equipment	5	4	3	2	1
2	This clinic's physical facilities are visually appealing	5	4	3	2	1
3	The clinic's employees are very well dressed and appear neat	5	4	3	2	1
4	The appearance of the physical facilities of the clinic is in keeping with the type of services provided	5	4	3	2	1
5	When the clinic promises to do something by a certain time, it does it	5	4	3	2	1
6	When customers have problems, the clinic is sympathetic and reassuring	5	4	3	2	1
7	The clinic is dependable	5	4	3	2	1
8	The clinic provides its services at the time, it promises to do so	5	4	3	2	1
9	The clinic keeps its records accurately	5	4	3	2	1
10	The clinic does not tell customers exactly when services will be performed	5	4	3	2	1
11	You do not receive prompt service from the employees of the clinic	5	4	3	2	1

S. No.	Items	SA	A	N	D	SD
12	The clinic's employees don't always have to be willing to help customers	5	4	3	2	1
13	Employees of the clinic are too busy to respond to customer requests promptly	5	4	3	2	1
14	You trust the employees of the clinic	5	4	3	2	1
15	You feel safe in your transactions with the clinic employees	5	4	3	2	1
16	The clinic employees are polite	5	4	3	2	1
17	The clinic employees get adequate support from the clinic to do their jobs well	5	4	3	2	1
18	The clinic does not give customers individual attention	5	4	3	2	1
19	Employees of the clinic do not give customers personal attention	5	4	3	2	1
20	Employees of the clinic do not know what the needs of their customers are	5	4	3	2	1
21	The clinic does not have your best interest at heart	5	4	3	2	1
22	The clinic has operating hours convenient to all their customers	5	4	3	2	1

PART 'D'

You have to put a Tick [√] mark in the appropriate option as per your opinion.

** Here SA=strongly agree; A=agree; N= Neutral; D=disagree and SD=strongly disagree.

ACCOUNTABILITY

S. No.	Items	SA	A	N	D	SD
1	In this diagnostic centre, the lab technicians possess the requisite qualifications to perform their tasks.	5	4	3	2	1
2	In this diagnostic centre, the pathologists possess the requisite qualifications to perform their tasks.	5	4	3	2	1
3	In case of any error, I have heard/experienced that this diagnostic centre takes responsibility for its actions.	5	4	3	2	1
4	In case of any error, I have heard/experienced that this diagnostic centre run the test, again free of cost (in case of any discrepancy).	5	4	3	2	1
5	In case of any error, I have heard/experienced that this diagnostic centre conducts a thorough enquiry to find out the cause behind the error.	5	4	3	2	1
6	I usually get my test done at the pre-scheduled time.	5	4	3	2	1
7	I usually get my test reports delivered on time.	5	4	3	2	1
8	I usually get timely reminders for my tests to be done afterwards.	5	4	3	2	1
9	This diagnostic centre has a proper grievance redressal system for its clients.	5	4	3	2	1
10	I have heard that the report generated by this diagnostic centre is authentic and reliable.	5	4	3	2	1
11	I usually get justifiable reasons for the actions performed by the diagnostic centre for any particular test.	5	4	3	2	1
12	This diagnostic centre follows the requisite protocols for all diagnoses and tests.	5	4	3	2	1
13	This diagnostic centre uses the latest technology prevalent in the relevant healthcare diagnostic industry for all the diagnoses and tests.	5	4	3	2	1
14	I find staff members of the diagnostic centre involved in distracting activities and other unproductive behaviour.	5	4	3	2	1

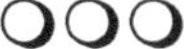

www.ingramcontent.com/pod-product-compliance
Ingram Content Group UK Ltd.
Pitfield, Milton Keynes, MK11 3LW, UK
UKHW062008290726
14090UKWH00022B/1447